Medical Disclaimer

The author does not guarantee any products or recommendations in this book will provide you with the same benefits other people have achieved. You should seek a doctor and do your own research to determine if any of the products or recommendations made by the author in this book will work for you.

While the author has made every effort to provide accurate product names and other information available at time of publication, neither the author nor the publisher assumes responsibility for errors or changes occurring after publication. Additionally, the author has no control over products or websites associated with the products listed in this book or the content of those websites.

This book is sold with the understanding that neither the author nor the publisher is engaged in rendering any legal, accounting, financial, medical, employment, or any other professional advice. If legal, accounting, financial, medical, employment, or any other professional advice is required, the services of a competent professional in those areas should be sought by you. The author and publisher shall have neither liability or responsibility to any person, company, or entity with respect to any loss or damage caused either directly or indirectly by the concepts, ideas, products, information, or suggestions presented in this book. By reading this book, you agree to be bound by the statements above.

Foods Making You Fat, Unhealthy, and Unhappy:

Your Personal Roadmap to Fix Problems Doctors Cannot

Book Three of the Lose Weight and Regain Health Series

Dr. Dale Heil

The Lose Weight and Regain Health Series in Order:

Is Pollution Making You Fat? Stop Toxins from Creating Fat

The Psychology Behind Eating: Scientifically Proven Mind Games to Lose Weight and Keep It Off

Foods Making You Fat, Unhealthy, and Unhappy: Your Personal Roadmap to Fix Problems Doctors Cannot

Arthritis, Pain Syndromes, and Feeling Older Than You Should: Your Personalized Path to Stop Pain

Receive a FREE Gift!

Building a relationship with my readers is the absolute best thing about writing. I love to send newsletters with details on new releases, special offers, and other bits related to the Lose Weight and Regain Health Series so we can build that relationship.

Get a FREE copy with email signup of the eBook *Modified Mediterranean Diet: Your Bridge to a Slimmer, Healthier Body That Looks and Feels Younger* by going to

https://dl.bookfunnel.com/l6yme0m6pl

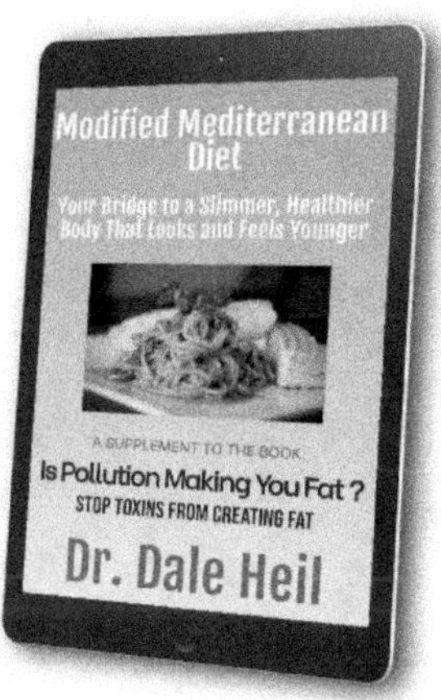

ALSO,

You can get the first chapter of the second book of this series, *The Psychology Behind Eating: Scientifically Proven Mind Games to Lose Weight and Keep It* Off where we look at using psychology to guide your mind to changing your eating habits that are easy, fun, and desirable.

That will be at the end of this book… and it's FREE

CONTENTS

Introduction

In the first book of this series, *Is Pollution Making You Fat? Stop Toxins from Creating Fat* we showed how environmental pollution and toxins lead to the establishment of vicious cycles of fat production and how to cure this situation. Now we will discuss how to determine what the healthiest foods are for your body because that differs from person to person.

Without knowing what you should eat, and what foods you should avoid based upon your particular bodily makeup, you can never realize the best health you can achieve. We will go over the means you can use to achieve your optimal level of health in an easy, step-by-step process.

As we go through this information, I will mention several resources you will need to achieve the goals you set for yourself. Don't worry. You can simply go to my website at WWW.DEHEIL.com where I have everything listed for you to make things easy. I will put that URL at the end of this book also to make it doubly easy for you. For right now, let's get you the information you need to eat the right foods to get your body in the best shape it's been in for years.

Now, let's look at how you can learn how to eat the foods your body wants and avoid the ones that will do it harm. This is important for several reasons. Eating the wrong foods will create inflammation in your body, making you look like a water balloon. It's not fat, but people mistake it for being overweight. Plus, inflammation creates pain in your body that may easily preclude you from wanting to move and enjoy life. Then there is the aspect of creating dangerous situations like high blood pressure, which further propels you down the path of ill health and disability.

Those things are not good, and you want to make sure you are eating the correct foods for your body so you can enjoy life to the fullest while looking great.

You may think you know the answer based on what you've read or heard in the popular media. I beg to differ from your preconceived notions because there is no cookie cutter diet that will work for everyone. There are simply too many variables unique to you. You look like no one else in this world. Your DNA differs from everyone else's on Earth. And your body is distinctive in what foods will benefit it so it stays healthy and which ones will produce sinister problems that slowly rob you of your precious health.

But just what is true health?

True health is when all your organs and systems are operating at the peak of their efficiency. It is a lot more than the mere absence of disease, though that is the way most people look at it. There are no set foods or groups of foods that when consumed will work for everyone, that's why the perfect diet has not yet been found. Did you ever wonder why there are so many diets and diet books floating around? Now you know the reason. None of them are optimized for the individual. It takes some work to figure out what foods are the best for you so follow the step-by-step process I will outline so you can easily figure out what foods are best for you and which ones you must avoid to regain and maintain true health.

Did you ever notice how truly healthy people have a certain "glow" about them that makes them attractive from the inside out? You often see it in young people before years of eating the wrong foods makes them look worn out and haggard. Persistently eating the wrong foods for your body will assure you continue down that road to self-destruction. On the other hand, there are some older people who just seem to radiate energy. Those are the ones who are eating foods that more closely match what their body wants them to be eating.

True health is easy to lose and hard to regain, but, with proper guidance and a little self-determination, true health can be relatively easy to maintain once you figure out which foods to eat and the ones to avoid. And you should avoid the foods that are bad for you. Treat them as though they are poison because that's what they are to your bodily systems.

Enough talking. Let's begin our discussion by having you look at the state of your body by making a list of symptoms you are currently plagued by.

Why should you do that?

Well, this is an important step in being able to monitor the internal workings of your body continually so you can make corrections when you stray from the foods you've proven to be beneficial to your personal health. Do not skip this step. You may be able to identify and correct problems that have plagued you for a long time.

Are you ready to have an eye-opening experience? Let's begin!

Oh! But first we must learn about canaries. Canaries? Like the birds? Yes, the birds. Read on to learn how you can use this fun and whimsical analogy to keep you healthy.

Chapter Two

Canary in the Mineshaft

Do you remember the old story of miners taking a canary into the mineshaft with them?

It was a primitive but very effective early warning device. Since the canary was so much smaller than a man it would be the first to succumb to the invisible, poisonous gases that can build up in a mine.

If the canary fell dead from its perch, the miners would take the hint and vacate the mine posthaste.

This concept may be primitive, but it is still useful in several ways. United States troops used chickens placed in cages on the front of their vehicles during the invasion of Iraq. They feared that nerve gas and biological weapons used by the Iraqi army could kill from five to ten thousand U.S. troops in the first few weeks of the war. The chickens were to be an early warning device, indicating the presence of these horrible substances.

Luckily, even though there were nerve agents found in captured shells gathered from the battlefield, none of these devilish weapons were deployed. The chickens probably survived, at least until a field-expedient chef got hold of them when the troops finally reached Baghdad.

You will use this concept of "a canary in the mineshaft" to monitor your personal health so you can use any symptoms you once had as an early warning device.

There are no blanket statements that can be made about how you are supposed to eat. Everyone is a unique individual and your body demands specific foods that work with it and for you to avoid the foods that work against it. That's why we will go through an extensive process (extensive, but easy, you'll see) to determine your canaries.

Canaries are a fun and whimsical concept I came up with that is based upon monitoring the symptoms you are suffering from and then see which ones disappear or reduce in intensity after you make the correct dietary changes for your individual body.

If you revert to your old eating habits, these canary symptoms will reappear to remind you in very certain terms that you must get back to the foods your body demands. That will keep you looking great, feeling tremendous, and being the best you've ever been.

Canaries in this discussion were designed to be fun and whimsical, but they are very serious tools we can use to keep ourselves on the right track regardless of whether our goal is to keep weight off after we lose it, look as young and vibrant as possible, or to improve our outlook on life. Of course, you can do all three, and your personal canaries will help you do it.

After completing your liver detoxification process as I discuss in the first book of this series, *Is Pollution Making You Fat? Stop Toxins from Creating Fat* showing you how it is almost impossible to take weight off and keep it off without rejuvenating your liver, it was suggested that this detoxification process may also ease some of the nagging health problems you have been suffering from for years. Well, now we are taking this concept to the next step by making a list of the health problems that disappear because of the changes in your eating habits you will make, relating them to your diet and not to a congested liver. When any health problem disappears, it is now elevated to the lofty status of being one of your "canaries."

Assuming you have followed the suggestions in that book and detoxified your liver, now you must determine which foods are beneficial for your unique body and which ones are detrimental to it.

Here is the process in an abbreviated form, so you have some information to get your mind around what you will be doing.

You will record your pre-dietary change symptom list so you can then make a comparison between it and after you make the suggested dietary changes. After you have your symptom list in hand, you'll change your diet, eating only food items beneficial to you and avoid detrimental ones. You will continue this for a few weeks.

After eating only beneficial foods for a few weeks, you are ready to make a before and after comparison that will reflect any reduction in your symptoms brought about by your dietary changes. This will be evidence that the changes in your eating habits resulted in positive changes in your health status.

What dietary changes will you have to make to ease some of your symptoms? Don't worry. I will give you a step-by-step process to determine your optimal foods to eat.

When we were looking at potential changes that may take place with liver detoxification, we looked at common symptoms people commonly suffer from such as allergies, hemorrhoids, varicose veins, skin conditions like eczema, dark circles under the eyes, chronic constipation, gas or bloating, heartburn, and binge eating. The list of symptoms you will look at extends far beyond these.

You will want to note any changes in your body, as they will be very important for you to monitor throughout your entire lifetime to maintain your optimal health. For example, if you notice certain symptoms returning after they had improved, your "canary" is showing signs of trouble. Usually, that's from allowing your poor eating habits to slip slowly back into your life.

This is a common occurrence. When people are feeling better and life is good, they forget what they did that got them to that point. The return of your canaries is a stark reminder that your diligence has been slipping and you must get back on track with your proper eating habits.

If, after reestablishing your proper eating habits, your canary resuscitates (i.e., your canary symptoms disappear again), you know you are doing a good job of restoring your proper eating habits.

This is a tremendous time to play around and once again prove to yourself that what you are doing is working. I cover this in much greater detail in my *The Psychology Behind Eating: Scientifically Proven Mind Games to Lose Weight and Keep It Off* book so you can easily understand this powerful tool you can use to achieve your goals. This simple act of creating a symptom list is what can change your eating habits forever by simply giving you the motivation to do what is making you feel better. And it's super easy to do.

This may not seem like a big deal, but it is. It's an enormous deal. When you find something that is working for you want to reinforce those eating behaviors. It's smart to keep doing what is beneficial and not simply forget and slowly drift back into your old habits. That will lead you down a dismal path you really don't want to be on.

As I point out in that book, canaries allow the behavior modification principles of psychology to be applied in an accurate and methodical method. In other words, you are no longer guessing. You have solid proof of what works for you as an individual and what does not. You've proven to yourself you are feeling better, and we always choose to do what makes us happier.

By using these principles, you will stay motivated to maintain the healthy eating habits you have now proven to yourself to be highly beneficial to your health and wellbeing. If you lose weight with these dietary changes, you will want to make sure you keep that weight off and your canaries will help ensure you do exactly that.

When you feel good and life is going along splendidly, your eating habits are "out of sight, out of mind." However, your canaries bring them to the forefront to stare you in the face. That will motivate you to do what you know you should have been doing all along.

To make checking your canary a habit and something you do not forget to do, you should establish a set time and date each week to review your canary checklist. The first thing every Monday morning as you get ready to start your work week or any other day of the week that is significant in your schedule should be your established time to check your canary checklist. Make it a habit. It's one of the better habits you can have.

It is vital for you to have a written checklist. As you are changing your eating habits, note any improvements in the typical symptoms you normally suffer from. They may not all improve but be sure to note those that do. Those are your canaries and they're vitally important to your continued health and wellbeing.

Write each of your canaries and physically put a checkmark behind each when you do your weekly evaluation. If you don't go through the physical act of checking it off your list, it is too easy for you to just skim over them and fall back into your old habits.

Remember, these are lifelong changes you are trying to establish. You want to be healthier and slimmer, and that is a lifelong program. The last thing you want is to improve your health, then go back to your old eating habits that allow your healthier body to slip back into ill health. Once you slip, it's difficult getting back into your good habits.

That's what happens with people who do not keep tabs on their canaries. It's not what healthy, successful people do so change your habits to stay where you want to be with your health.

Only by consistently and thoroughly monitoring the internal functions of your body via the external expression of symptoms can you make lifelong changes in your health, keep the accumulation of body fat in check, and maintain healthier eating habits.

Canaries offer an easy, inexpensive, non-invasive, and effective way to monitor the functioning of your internal organs. This concept is not new. Canaries are also used in many other aspects of the sciences, though they may not be called that.

Biologists use the "canary" concept of monitoring a target species to keep abreast of the health of that species' environment. For example, they may monitor the trout population in a stream to keep a watch on the health of that stream.

Trout are very sensitive to changes in their environment. They are likely to be one of the first creatures living in a stream to die if the water quality or temperature changes. Trout have a narrow range of environmental parameters they need to survive. Change any of those parameters and the trout dies before other species begin dying.

The biologists can watch for dead trout or a decrease in the number of trout in that stream to determine if something has changed in that watercourse. It is then an arduous task to find out what those changes are and correct them, if possible. This method is often used to monitor pollution, such as mine acid drainage or other habitat destroying conditions, so all aquatic life is not destroyed.

If scientists are using canaries, you should use them as well. Canaries can help you stay healthy, and health is more valuable than all gold and treasure.

Chapter Three

Your Canaries Will Guide You

As a health care practitioner discussing health and diet, I prefer to see health-related issues in terms of having a healthy, correctly functioning body because of proper eating habits or not. Keeping the issue as clear as possible makes things easier to understand. This helps direct people from a state of ill health to improved health.

We're going to relate your health status and the problems you are experiencing directly to your eating habits and the foods you consume. In this way, you can shift the focus of your efforts toward the positive aspects of eating the foods that are correct for you and avoid those that are not.

Everyone wants to know how they should eat to lose weight and stay healthy. Whether they follow a healthy eating plan is another question, but everyone always wants information whether they do what they're supposed to or not.

Most of you reading this book may be interested in losing weight, in addition to being healthy. That's a good thing! But there is more to being healthy than just looking good at the beach.

But how do you know which of the multitude of diets floating around out there are likely to make and keep you healthy? Each new diet book that comes out makes that claim, but will the diets they espouse truly work for you?

Maybe not.

There are too many unknown variables to determine if any diet will be a good one for you or not. We're going to narrow down some of those unknown variables and make them known entities you can prove to yourself are working the way you want them to.

What works for one person may not work for you. That's why you must put some effort into finding out what your specific food needs are... and how to avoid the foods that seem innocent but in reality are jeopardizing your ability to obtain maximal health. Don't worry, it's not a difficult or labor-intensive procedure. As you will soon find out, the route you will embark on is not only fun, but extremely informative.

Canned, planned, and one-size-fits-all diets won't work for you because they were not tailored specifically for you. We're going to outline a process by which you can determine what foods are good for you and which ones you should avoid.

As you go through the process of discovering which foods your body wants (which makes it thrive) and the foods it does not want (which will give you some sign it is not happy with those foods) you will want to keep two lists. One list will be of the foods you should eat, and the other list is those foods you should avoid. Keep these lists in a safe place. Make a few copies of them and stash them in different places because you will refer to them often as you create or change recipes using the foods that will make your body thrive.

Before we get into all that, let's define what being healthy truly means.

Most people think that if they are not flat on their back in bed, in the hospital, or suffering from recurring episodes of pain and suffering, then they are healthy. That's not what we're talking about here.

Many people feel great until the point they fall over dead from a massive coronary. Were they healthy the few seconds before crushing chest pain snuffed their life out? No, they weren't. They felt good, but they were not healthy.

For this discussion, you'll want to define health as having all your bodily systems operating at 100%. That's nice, but how are you supposed to know if your body is working correctly or not? And if not, to what degree is it out of whack?

Here's how you are going to find what foods work for you and which work against you. Remember, you want to get your bodily systems operating as close to 100% as you can get them. Here's the formula to figure out your customized eating plan.

Begin by making a list of all the symptoms you have (that's the first step in making your canary list) as well as take a few measurements of various body parts. This may be more difficult than you imagine, but it's vitally important for you to find healthy eating habits that are custom made for you.

Make time to sit down and think. Ten minutes is the bare minimum of time you should devote to this exercise. It may take much longer than that, and that's OK. It's your personal list. Take all the time you need to make it as complete as you can.

It is usually best to find a quiet place that is comfortable, though sitting alone on the train commuting to work may work just as well for you. You must be able to concentrate without interruptions wherever you choose to sit to compile this list. This can be done anywhere, but you must be able to think, concentrate, and record what you come up with.

You'll need something to record your observations. That could be as old-fashioned as a pencil and paper or as modern as a digital file on your computer or phone. It doesn't matter as long as you can easily retrieve the information at later dates.

Be as observant and picky as you can be while compiling your list. Begin at the top of your head and work your way down your body. Is your hair thinning? Or is it super thick? Lackluster? Oily? Dry? Falling out faster than you can grow new hair?

Next body part down is your scalp. Do you have any problems with your scalp? Does it itch? Do you get flakes of dry skin floating off the top of your head?

Slide farther down and think about your eyes and ears. Do you have any problems with them? Please. Don't get hung up on whether you think your ears are too big or your eyes aren't the color you wish they were. Be honest but real when making this list. It's important.

How about your habits? Do you sleep well? Do you sleep all the time and can't wake up enough to function throughout the day? How about your mental health? Are you nervous? Aggressive? Blasé toward the pleasures of life? Pay close attention to all aspects of your life and record them by putting one item on each line of your paper or on your computer or phone.

Think about these things and try to determine what is not "normal" when compared to other people. All too many times, people learn to live with symptoms that may show something going on inside of them they thought they had no control over. As it may turn out, you could be able to improve or even reverse some of these symptoms that may have been with you for many years. That's why you must be able to retrieve this information, so you can make comparisons to see if improvements are being made as you change your diet for the better. In this manner, you will customize your diet specifically for you by using the information your body is giving you.

If you cannot think of what symptoms you may suffer from, use a list such as that found at https://my.standardprocess.com/Products/Literature/Systems-Survey-Form This is the Standard Process Symptom Survey used by doctors to determine what nutrition a person needs. You will not be using it for those purposes, but instead, you can use it to jog your memory in case there are any symptoms you forgot about but want to add to the list you are making. You can find this survey in other places by doing an Internet search for it if this link ever stops working. It's very popular, so you should have no problem finding it if you search for it.

After you have completed your list of symptoms, make a few copies with just the list of symptoms because in the next step you will rate the severity of your symptoms. These can be physical copies on paper or digital copies stored on your computer. You will use this list repeatedly, but you do not want to see how you rated each of the symptoms on previous occasions.

After you have your list of symptoms and made a few copies, it's time to rate them as to the severity of each one. Use a scale from 1 to 10. One is where the symptoms are very mild and hardly worth mentioning. Ten is where it is severe and seriously impacting your life. Make sure you put the date on each of these copies as you rate each of your symptoms. That will allow you to stay organized so you can see trends from one date to the next.

Please do not confuse this symptom list with your canaries. Your list of symptoms is simply that, a list. Only after those symptoms improve do they get put on your canary list. Those are the symptoms you want to monitor forever to make sure they never worsen or come back if they have totally resolved and disappeared.

Is that all? Make a symptom list? No problem, right?

Well, it may not be the only thing you want to do. When you eat the correct foods and avoid the ones that are not good for you, it may change the size and shape of your body. Therefore, take some measurements of specific areas of your body so you can monitor them as well.

When measuring body parts, it is easiest to use a flexible cloth ruler or tailor measuring tape like they use for sewing clothing. This tool allows you to take measurements accurately around body parts that a straight ruler or rigid tape measure will not.

If you aren't happy with your belly, measure it, but make sure you find a spot what you can find again to measure later. That means you may have to find the tops of your hipbones, measure up a few inches, and then take your measurement. With all these types of measurements, it is always best to begin a known distance from a bony prominence. Otherwise, you may be off by a few inches if you try measuring only soft tissues (that's that they're called in medical terminology, it has nothing to do with how "soft" your belly may currently be).

Make sure you record the bony prominence you are measuring from how high above or below that prominence you are taking the measurement, and what the exact measurement turns out to be. If you are measuring the circumference of your thighs, pick a bony spot on your knee, measure up a specific distance above that spot, and take your measurement. The same with your arms or any other part you want to monitor. Just remember to record all the pertinent information so you can repeat the measurement with the greatest accuracy possible.

You can do the same with the flexibility of our joints. People who have arthritis, or at least arthritic symptoms, can move their joints as far as they can go. Take a measurement the best you can and record it on your symptom list. Later, you will make a comparison between this first recorded measurement and subsequent ones.

There are specialized tools called goniometers you can buy to measure the flexibility of joints, but that level of accuracy may not be necessary. Guessing at how many degrees your joints are moving or comparing one limb to the other to get a percentage of how much motion it is lacking is usually sufficient.

Does that make sense? Good. Now, let's move on to the steps you must take to pare down the list of foods that will be good for you and those that are not.

Chapter 4

Beginning Your Healthy Eating Plan

Once you have your list of symptoms and how severe they are, you can begin seeking out the foods you should eat and those you should be avoiding. There are a few steps to this process, so be patient.

To begin this process, you must read the book entitled Eat Right 4 Your Type by Dr. Peter J. D'Adamo. I have a link to it from my website found at WWW.DEHEIL.com to make it easy for you to find and to assure you get the correct book. This book is easy to read and will help you find the foods that are highly beneficial for you to eat, the ones that are neutral, and those you should avoid based on your blood type.

Naturally, you will need to know your blood type to use the information in this book. If you don't know your blood type, check with your doctor. A free way to find out is by donating blood to your local blood bank. They always type the blood when they receive it. Besides, donating blood will help someone in trouble and in need of a blood transfusion. It's a win-win situation, for sure. They'll be happy to tell you what your blood type is, and they often give you a laminated card with the information on it so you do not forget.

But you don't want to read another book, right? You're reading this one and you want to know all the secrets to losing weight and being healthy from this one source. That's understandable but you're going to have to read Dr. D'Adamo's book because it is a wealth of information and way too much to explain here, though we will cover a bit about why the information in Dr. D'Adamo's book is so vital.

All the information in this process I am laying out for you is already out there, often in books that have been available for decades, but it's scattered all over. I am going to point you in the right direction, then give you the step-by-step procedure to bring all this information together so it is usable. Weeding out misinformation and then organizing the proper steps to take and in which sequence you should take them will give you what you want to know.

Think of finding which foods are good for you to eat and which ones are causing you harm as being like an onion. First, you peel off the first layer, then you can see the second layer, but you cannot see the third layer until you peel the second one away, and so on. It's a very interesting process that is fascinating to see unfold.

Reading Dr. D'Adamo's book is only the first step in weeding out the bad foods that are causing you a ton of problems. There are other steps you must take to fine-tune what your body wants and doesn't want in it, and they are just as easy as this one, so don't get discouraged. The results you will reap are well worth the effort you expend.

Why are there multiple steps involved in this food-discovery process? It's because each one digs deeper into discovering which foods are causing you problems and which ones are helpful to you as an individual.

As Dr. D'Adamo points out, the wrong food FOR YOU can cause inflammation. Inflammation inside your body can make you look and feel like a water balloon. Don't believe it? Shake any area of fat on your body. Is it solid or does it jiggle like a bowl full of Jello? If it does, you have inflammation and you basically are a water balloon. That should make you feel good. If you eat the correct foods based upon your blood type, and avoid those that cause inflammation FOR YOU, then you can easily rid yourself of the fluid that is accumulating in your bodily tissues.

The inflammation inside you is much more insidious and dangerous than just making you look flabby. It causes plaquing in your arteries and makes your heart pump stronger to push blood through all those congested tissues. That raises your blood pressure, which is not good. So, don't ignore the importance of the foods you eat.

If you're consuming the wrong food, regardless of how little of it you eat, it can be very detrimental to your health. Besides, inflammation is basically water, and water weighs approximately eight pounds per gallon. That's a lot of weight you may carry around on your body that you really don't need to. By reducing the inflammation in your body, you can then have a more realistic idea of what is fat and what is fluid.

After trying this diet for a few months, you may find your body type changing. Instead of being soft, you may notice you are getting firmer. If you find it is true, and it makes you happier, it's a good thing, right?

Don't forget to write it down, because now it's one of your canaries. Yes, it is very subjective, but it is still a canary.

Someone with a different blood type than yours may do well eating other foods that are detrimental to you and vice versa. This is a highly individualistic undertaking and is the reason all the "wonder diets" do not work for everyone.

You've noticed that, right? A friend tried a certain diet that is being touted in the popular media as the best thing for humankind and they are doing fantastically on it. Then you try it, and it is horrible for you. You begin wondering what's wrong with you. Why is that diet working for everyone else, but not for you? That's because that diet had foods in it that more closely matched someone with a different blood type than you have.

Conversely, you may have found the diet you do very well on, but your friends do not. They end up being disillusioned with what you were suggesting to them, and you feel bad because they did not do as well as you did on that diet. It strains relationships, and you don't need that in your life as well. Now you know why that phenomenon occurs with one person doing well on a certain diet while others do not. It's your differing blood types (and maybe other factors which we will delve into later) that give you differing results.

Find out your blood type, read Dr. D'Adamo's book, and do what it says. This is the first step in the process of you working toward a new way of eating and loving life.

Commit to eating the right foods for your blood type for two weeks. Please look upon the foods on your list of foods to avoid due to your specific blood type as poison. Do not eat them, not even a little.

This is not the type of diet you want to "cheat" on. It will sabotage your success and cause major problems. Remember the poison analogy I just made? A little poison can harm you, as can the foods that are wrong for your blood type. Besides, cheating will mess up the data you need to apply the principles of behavior modification as outlined in the book *The Psychology Behind Eating: Scientifically Proven Mind Games to Lose Weight and Keep It Off.*

Since I mentioned the second book in this book series, let me explain how I organized this information. The second book, as I mentioned, is the psychology book. That book is necessary because our mind dictates how successful we will be at losing weight and then keeping it off. Why lose all that weight just to put it all back on again? And maybe add a few pounds just for good measure? It's what usually happens with people's weight loss efforts, and I wrote this book to avoid that from happening to you.

The third book of the series is the one you are currently reading. The first two books were for people who only want to learn how to lose weight and keep it off. If that is your only goal, then the first two books are enough for you. I wrote this third book for people who want to be as healthy as they can be, or those who have terrible health problems they want to reduce or even eliminate.

The fourth book of the series is for people who have very serious health issues that are gravely affecting their lives. It is called *Arthritis, Pain Syndromes, and Feeling Older Than You Should: Your Personalized Path to Stop Pain.*

Each of these books takes the reader further into determining which foods they should eat, and which ones are detrimental to their health. I wrote them in a series because everyone may not want to follow the process to the end because they are happy stopping somewhere along the way. By setting this book series up in this manner, readers can get the results they crave and stop when they want to.

Now, back to the business at hand.

Great! You made it through two weeks of eating according to the blood type diet as explained by Dr. D'Amato and it's time to use one of your symptom lists to record how you're doing. Make sure you use one of the lists that does not have numbers on it from when you initially rated the intensity of your symptoms. You don't want that information tainting your evaluation from today.

Always put the date at the top of each symptom list so you can keep track of when you rated your symptoms. You want the rating part to be blank to avoid seeing how you were feeling previously, but you want to know exactly what date you filled out that form so you can look back at our records to see your progress.

If you can see a reduction in your symptoms, that's great! It means eating right for your blood type is working. If you don't see any reduction in your symptoms, that's alright. It's early and you still have time.

But what do you do now?

You have some fun by dietarily crashing yourself. Take two days (the weekend works well since you can justify eating all kinds of tasty things when you're out enjoying yourself) and consume all the things you've been avoiding for the last two weeks.

Yahoo! Fun! Right?

It's all great fun until Monday (the third day). This is the day you use another one of your symptom lists to see what effect those foods you'd been avoiding for the past two weeks have had on you. Compare the ratings of symptom severity you took before crashing yourself (In this scenario, that would have been Friday since you're doing this over the weekend) and those you get on Monday (the third day of your crash eating).

Are you confused yet? Don't worry, I'll give you a summary at the end of this chapter that will make this entire process easy to work your way through.

What most people find is that their symptoms were reduced on Friday (just before the dietary crash) and they felt better. Then, on Monday, after crashing their diet, they feel much worse. That's the magic of behavior modification. People gravitate toward things that make them feel good (are pleasurable) and avoid things that make them feel bad. In this case, it reinforces the fact you were feeling better when you were not eating the foods that are bad for you (assuming you saw such a reduction in symptoms or at least the intensity of the symptoms, which you should).

Don't expect changes in your eating behavior to occur overnight. However, after you realize how good you feel when eating the correct foods for your blood type and how crummy you feel when eating the foods you should avoid, you will naturally gravitate toward healthier eating to keep yourself feeling better.

Behavior modification is a powerful tool so you may as well use it to your advantage. This is simply the psychology of eating. Learn to control your environment instead of allowing it to control you.

Some improvements in how you feel may have been difficult to quantify before applying the blood type diet as outlined by Dr. D'Adamo. But afterward, especially after following a structured program to monitor them, you can usually see a difference. It may be an enormous difference or it may only be a subtle difference, but there is almost always a difference if you accurately recorded and monitored the symptoms on your list.

Here is a phenomenon we've not covered yet.

That's the situation where a food item is supposed to be good for you but isn't. For instance, they may tout a certain food as being good for everyone's health, but that does not mean it is good for you as an individual. Someone else may have tremendous results with a specific diet or food item, but you don't. This system will allow you to find out what works for you and you alone.

I once had a patient who we will call Roseanne. She did exceptionally well on the ketogenic diet. I mean, she did really well. Roseanne lost a lot of weight, felt great, began a rigorous training program and was doing fantastically with it.

At least most of the time. There was just something that wasn't 100% right with that diet and her body, but she didn't know what it was.

Eventually, we were able to trace the discord to coconut oil. That oil is a huge part of the ketogenic diet and does well for most people. It was even one of the foods on Roseanne's highly beneficial list as outlined in Dr. D'Adamo's book, but it wasn't working for her. Further testing (which we will cover in greater detail shortly) revealed she had a sensitivity to coconut oil.

Who would have thought?

Once Roseanne stopped consuming coconut oil, everything went splendidly for her and continues to do so. She merely had to be a detective and take additional steps to find the one food that did not agree with her body (it could have been other foods, but it wasn't, and testing proved it). It's that unique thing about each of our bodies being different and the need to discover what is good for us as individuals or not.

Once you clear out the items on your list of foods to avoid based upon your blood type, it will make the foods that are supposedly beneficial for you but aren't to stand out. If you find a food item that causes you problems, make a note about it on your symptom list. At that point, you can add that food item to your personal avoid list and don't eat the stuff.

Summary Up to This Point

We've gone over a lot of information, so let's take a moment to summarize it all up to this point. A summary will help you keep everything straight in your mind. For a more in-depth overview of the process to find which foods you should eat, and which ones are causing you harm, you can peruse the *Executive Summary and Workbook* I wrote. That tome puts every step one after the other and not only keeps it all organized for you, but it also gives you the opportunity to determine how far you want to go in finding the perfect diet for your unique body.

1) Make a list of your symptoms and record body measurements (including circumference of body parts and range of motion of joints, if applicable.) Remember to make copies without the numbers showing so you can rate your symptoms at later dates without seeing what you put down previously.

2) Read Eat Right 4 Your Type by Dr. Peter J. D'Adamo and set up your eating plan based upon your blood type. If you do not know your blood type, contact your doctor or donate blood if you are eligible to do so.

3) Eat only the foods on your beneficial or neutral lists, consuming mostly the beneficial foods and less of the neutrals. Completely stay away from the foods on your avoid list, treating them like poison.

4) Two weeks later, go through your symptom survey again, rating each symptom as to how intense it is currently.

5) Have fun and crash yourself for two days eating all the things you've eaten all your life, making sure you eat lots of the foods on your avoid list. (Yes, you will binge on the foods you are supposed to avoid. You want to see how much they negatively affect you so gorge yourself on them!)

6) On the third day, after two days of crashing yourself, go through your symptom survey again rating each symptom how intense it is currently. If the severity of your symptoms went up compared to only two or three days previously, then you have proof of your newfound diet positively affecting those symptoms.

7) Get back on the Eat Right 4 Your Type regimen again and don't look back except to rate your symptoms every few weeks to see if more of those stubborn symptoms are fading away as time goes on.

Food Sensitivity Testing

Remember the story of Roseanne I told you about a few paragraphs ago? Well, we determined coconut oil was not working for her by performing a food sensitivity test.

Yes, I know. It is something else you must do to find the foods that are good for you and are not bad for you. But food sensitivity tests offer you an opportunity to fine-tune your list of foods to avoid.

But what is a food sensitivity? And is it different from a food allergy?

Well, a food sensitivity is a delayed non-life-threatening immune response to a specific food by the individual person. They usually discover it by doing a blood test for the reactivity of IgG antibodies (remember the IgG part, it will be important in a moment). Common symptoms may include gastrointestinal symptoms such as bloating, headaches, and an entire litany of other symptoms too many to mention.

A food allergy, on the other hand, is an immediate, potentially life-threatening immune response to a specific food. They usually confirm it with a skin prick test or a blood test for IgE antibodies (the difference is in the IgE of the food allergy as opposed to the IgG of a food sensitivity). Common symptoms may include coughing, wheezing, flushed skin, rash, hives, an itchy sensation in the mouth, or swelling of the face, tongue, and lips.

For this discussion, we are only interested in food sensitivities and how they affect your body. Remember, this is finding the perfect list of foods for you to eat based upon your unique individuality (nothing is perfect, I know, but we will get as close to perfection for you as we can). Food sensitivity testing fine tunes what you have already done and proven to yourself to be beneficial for you via your symptom list. Besides, you're worth it and you deserve the best, so do it.

These tests are not cheap, but they are very helpful, and it's all relative. If you are miserable because of the problems you are experiencing by eating the wrong food, wouldn't you be happy to spend a few dollars to be rid of those annoying (and possibly health depleting) symptoms? Isn't it worth it to move freely without pain?

Oh, you didn't know that eating the wrong foods can give you mobility problems? Well, I wrote an entire book on this topic. It's called *Arthritis, Pain Syndromes, and Feeling Older Than You Should: Your Personalized Path to Stop Pain.*

Let me tell you about James, a former patient of mine.

For decades, James had been suffering from pain between his shoulder blades, which then caused his neck to stiffen to the point of being unable to move his head. He'd seen a long line of chiropractors before ending up in my office. Most of the chiropractors had offered him relief of his symptoms, but only for a few days, then the pain and stiffness would slowly return until he could hardly move a week later. It was a vicious cycle of relief and the return of pain and disability he knew was coming a week later. James was miserable when that occurred, and he'd experienced that vicious cycle for so long he accepted it as the way his life would always be.

It looked like he was doomed to repeat the scenario he had become so accustomed to for the rest of his life until I suggested he go through the same program I suggested for you. After reading the book Eat Right 4 Your Type by Dr. Peter J. D'Adamo, he diligently followed the menu suggested by his blood type. It was a surprise to James that many of the problems on his symptom list cleared up or were reduced. Dishearteningly though, the pain between his shoulder blades that radiated up into his neck persisted, requiring his weekly chiropractic visit.

That's when we tried the food sensitivity test (I use the test by Everlywell, but there are others that may better suit you depending upon your preferences. I put a link to some of them on my website to make finding them easy for you.)

The food sensitivity test James took came back showing a moderate sensitivity to egg whites, egg yolks, and lamb. They separate the egg yolk from the egg whites because some people can have a sensitivity to one but not the other. In James's case, he was sensitive to both.

James did not eat lamb very often, but he kept a flock of chickens and had most of his life. Considering all the eggs he had readily available, it's not surprising he ate them every day, and he ate a lot of them.

It was hard for him to give up eating eggs, but he did. Shocking both of us, the pain and stiffness he'd been experiencing most of his life disappeared within a few weeks. The change in his health status was nothing short of phenomenal!

Naturally, I had to tell him to crash himself to see what happened. Sure enough, eating eggs for two days caused enough of the pain between his shoulder blades to return that he swore off eggs and still does not eat them. I called him a few months later, and he confirmed he was still avoiding eggs, had reduced the size of his chicken flock to a few select pets, and has not had a problem with pain between his shoulder blades since.

Does that sound strange? It is strange, but true. There are many physical problems arising from eating the foods you have a sensitivity to. There is no accurate list of these problems because each person is a unique individual and their body reacts differently to various foods.

Ask yourself, what foods are making you miserable or not allowing you to reach your optimal health? Isn't it worth it to follow the path to eating the correct foods that may make your life so much more enjoyable?

I put a list of a few of the food sensitivity tests on my website to make it easy for you to find one you like. They even make pet food and environmental intolerance tests for your pets if they are suffering from maladies their veterinarian cannot diagnose. Once again, these are tools to keep pets healthy and it seems they are way ahead of any available to keep people on the right track.

Detailed directions come with the food sensitivity test kits, so I will not go into that. However, I must stress that you follow those directions exactly. There is a reason they are so explicit in the directions and if you do not follow them precisely, you may expect less-than-perfect results from those tests. Just like the old saying about computers, "Garbage In, Garbage Out." If you give the laboratory a garbage sample of your blood, expect garbage information about it to come back to you.

If you give them contaminated or otherwise incomplete test kits to work with, you can, and should expect they cannot do the best job for you. Take the time to read the directions closely and do exactly what they say to get the best results. You'll be happy you did.

Now you know how to find the foods you should eat and those you should avoid as though they are poison. But what about the foods themselves? Are there differences in foods and should we be concerned about it? Yes, there are differences in foods and you must know about them if you are to get the most out of those you consume. Let's explore foods (which is always a popular topic) and how to choose the best foods to optimize your health.

Are Organic Vegetables Necessary?

It doesn't matter what your blood type is, there are always some foods in each of the major categories for people to choose from. One of those categories is fruits and vegetables. While the fruits and vegetables you should eat may vary from one blood type to the next, and your food sensitivity test may show up a few of them to avoid, if your fruits and vegetables are organically grown it can be an enormous factor in how your body reacts to them.

Does it matter whether the fruits and vegetables you eat are organically or chemically grown? Yes, it does. Let's explore why there is such a tremendous difference in the nutritional quality of the foods you consume.

Let's start with the vegetables themselves and discuss why organically grown veggies are always best. Period.

Yes, I know, you may not be able to afford organic vegetables and fruits, and there is no doubt they are more expensive than the ones grown in chemically fertilized fields. Regardless, if you are going to buy your produce at the grocery store, you should still know why organic is better.

I am not trying to be a vegetable snob by making such a statement. It is a fact that is very important to your health and wellbeing. There appear to be scientifically provable differences in the nutrient content of organically grown foods when compared to those raised with chemical fertilizers.

No big deal, you may think. Right?

Well, remember you are making your body healthier by assuring that your organs and the systems they control are operating at peak efficiency. To reach that end, you must eat a lot of raw vegetables and fruits to get the enzymes, phytonutrients, vitamins, and minerals that are only available from raw food sources. This isn't some nutty vegetarian, only eat "rabbit food" type of scheme. This is reality. Not your reality, but the reality of nature.

Raw vegetables and fruits must be a major portion of your daily food intake. Without the nutrients found in raw vegetables and fruits, consumed in sufficient quality and quantity, your bodily systems will never be truly healthy… and neither will you!

These are the nutrients your body needs every day to continue operating properly. Try running your automobile without gasoline or oil for an entire day. How far do you think you'll get? Your body operates on the same principle.

Remember, health and being slim go together. You'll never be as healthy as you can be if you do not eat the right foods to supply your body with the essential, let me repeat that, ESSENTIAL nutrients found in raw vegetables and fruits.

Organic foods offer more of the essential nutrients, of a quality sufficient to perform the tasks your body demands of them, than does chemically fertilized produce. Without nutrients of adequate quality and quantity consumed daily, your body cannot function correctly. Therefore, you do not stand a chance of getting as healthy as you can be if you do not do what your body demands.

Would you put inferior or watered-down gasoline into your car? Of course not. It wouldn't run correctly, and irreparable damage would occur to the mechanisms. But you're perfectly willing to do this to your body. Why?

OK, let's see if we can give you some information that will at least make you an informed consumer of food. What you do with that information is up to you.

Way back in 1939, it was espoused by the Cheshire Panel Committee that food grown with chemical fertilizers caused a deterioration of health in both humans and animals. While the public often speculates it is the deletion of pesticide and herbicide residues making organically grown foods better, it may be that these foods have a greater nutritional value because of elements in the soil and fertilizers used in organic farming.

Prior to World War II, there was no such thing as agricultural chemicals being used to grow vegetables. I have long suspected this may have been the case. When I viewed pictures of people from the WW II era, they are usually slender and well proportioned. They were built differently than people are today.

This is especially easy to visualize in the men of that era. These men were not gargantuan behemoths like so many of our young men today. They were muscular without being bulky and slender while lacking the unhealthy accumulation of body fat that is so prevalent today.

Look at photos with WWII servicemen posing bare-chested. You can find those images on the Internet, just take a few moments to search for them. Then compare it to pictures of today's servicemen. Note the difference in their build and muscle patterns. It's striking.

These differences are most likely because of several changes in our environment and not just the reduction of nutritional content in foods grown with chemical fertilizers. Though I will not rule out the major impact organically grown foods had on that generation, or the effects derived from the lack of quality foods influencing our current generation.

Regardless, there have been demonstrable declines in the mineral and vitamin content of fresh foods over the intervening decades.

A study by Worthington found organic crops had a higher nutrient content in more than half of the comparisons between organically grown and chemically fertilized foods.

That's important to know.

For those not familiar with organic farming methods, and do not know why they are superior to chemically grown foods, let's review the differences between the two.

Organic farming methods do not use pesticides or herbicides. In the United States, for a product to be called "organic" it must be grown in soil that has not been exposed to pesticides or herbicides for at least three years. To reduce damage caused by bugs and weeds, several alternative pest control methods are used.

Crop rotation, where different crops are grown in an area every other year, is used to reduce the opportunity for bugs and other pests to proliferate and damage crops. Rotating crops help avoid depleting the soil of vital minerals and nutrients. Growing the same crops, which demand the same nutrients from the soil from one growing season to the next quickly depletes the soil of those nutrients. By rotating crops, soil nutrient depletion is reduced. Certain crops are grown because they add nutrients to the soil as they grow. That's cool. Some plants take the nutrients out while others put them back in. Farmers just need to know which crops to grow at what time.

Organic farmers use cover crops to protect the soil from erosion. This avoids having nutrients washing away during rains. As cover crops grow, they protect the soil from nutrient depletion. Once grown, they can plow the cover crops into the soil to replenish nutrient content. Specific cover crops, when tilled into the soil, are called "green manure" because they restore nutrients to the soil.

They often augment green manure with other nutrient sources, such as aged manure from farm animals and plant wastes. Manure and other waste products are often composted, so they will more readily release their nutrients to the soil. Composting involves controlled rotting of waste materials to enhance desirable microbial action. The act of composting results in nutrient rich soil enhancements that are often referred to as "black gold" by organic gardeners.

All these organic farming practices restore organic material to the soil. Organic material, when reintroduced to the soil, preserves soil structure, and encourages the propagation of beneficial soil microorganisms. In this manner, soil nutrients are slowly released to the plants over a long period. That slow release of nutrients is desirable for proper plant nourishment.

In contrast, chemical fertilizers offer very few mineral substances for growing plants. Since chemical fertilizers are water soluble, they are only available to the growing plants for a short period before washing away during the next rain. At the time chemical fertilizers are applied to the soil, there is an overabundance of minerals available to growing plants. After a rain or lapse of a short period, the minerals dissipate. When using chemical fertilizers, soil structure and microorganism propagation is not encouraged, which hinders growth of the plants.

Soil structure and the quantity and quality of microorganisms in the soil have an enormous impact on the quantity of nutrients available to plants. Vegetables grown in soils containing substantial quantities of microorganisms have higher mineral content, and those are minerals your body desperately needs.

Several types of chemical fertilizers may even contain toxic heavy metals. That is dangerous because the heavy metals enter the soil and are absorbed by the plants. Upon eating the tainted vegetables, the heavy metals are transferred to you. That's not good and should be strenuously avoided.

The addition of chemical nitrogen fertilizers increases the absorption of any heavy metal toxins in the soil. Uh-Oh! A double whammy!

But does this really make a difference? Well, in one word, yes. It makes a vast difference.

Organically grown foods are always at least as nutritious as conventionally grown vegetables using chemical fertilizers (conventional for the last few decades, at least). In several instances, organic vegetables are more nutritious. Organic vegetables are never found to be less nutritious than their chemically grown counterparts.

Plus, they found the reproductive capability and resistance to infection in animals to be affected when they consumed conventionally grown chemically fertilized crops compared to organic. If this is happening in animals, it may happen in people as well.

That's important to remember.

A review of research compared antioxidant levels found in organic and chemically raised foods. In eighty-five percent of the foods studied, this review found the produce from organic farms having higher levels of antioxidants. Antioxidants are very good for you, and you want to consume a lot of them, so organic produce may be the way to go to assure you are getting everything you think you are in the foods you consume.

In this research review, the antioxidant levels of organic vegetables were thirty percent higher than those grown in chemically fertilized soils. That's very important since antioxidants reduce heart and arterial disease, slow the aging process, and they inhibit the reproduction of cancer cells. The increased antioxidant levels found in organically grown foods appear to make them worth the extra cost and effort.

The economics of striving for higher yields of crops per acre, and the quest for cheaper food, is largely to blame for the decline in the quality of our foods. While the quantity of food per acre has been increased by using chemical fertilizers, the nutritional food quality has suffered as evidenced by decreased quantities of nutrients in those foods.

They rarely identify this dilution of the quality of your food as a reason for the increasing incidence of people suffering from an unhealthy accumulation of body fat, but it should be. We have more food with fewer nutrients. It's almost like the "empty calories" syndrome found in fast foods where they are high in calories and low in nutrition.

This is an important concept for you to grasp because the reduction in the nutritional content of your foods may contribute to the establishment of an overloaded liver. That may contribute to an unhealthy accumulation of body fat and a slow decline in your overall health.

Because it is such a gradual decline in your health, you will not notice and may erroneously (and dangerously) think of the changes in your body as being "normal" or "a normal part of aging." It's not. It's your poor diet resulting in slowly declining health that can make your life miserable with illness and lead to a shorter life overall.

The deficient nutritional content of your foods may cause you to overeat. Your body monitors the quantity of nutrients you are consuming. Once you have consumed enough of the nutrients your body needs, your body signals you are full. You must remember that when your body is nutritionally satisfied, overeating and binge eating are greatly reduced or eliminated.

Make sure you start your day with nutrition packed foods, so you aren't tempted to eat more calories than you need later. Quality foods are well worth the time, effort, and/or expense.

If enzymes and other nutrients are not available in your food, your body will continue searching for food by making you hungry. Without essential nutrients, how can you expect your liver to detoxify toxins and expel them from your body or any other function of your body to operate correctly? Remember, enzymes and nutrients allow your liver to perform the vital function of detoxification.

But what are you supposed to do if you don't have access to organic vegetables or cannot grow your own? Well, you're stuck with what they sell at the local supermarket. They probably grew supermarket vegetables with chemical fertilizers unless labelled as being organically grown.

Don't fret over it. You have another avenue to make up the difference.

What's the solution? You must take organically grown whole food nutritional supplements. But they're expensive! Yes, but it's more costly to your body not to buy them.

Ask yourself, are you and your family worth it? Do you want to be healthy and have an acceptable amount of body fat or not? It's your choice.

Without the enzymes and nutrients quality foods in one form or the other contain, you will never achieve a healthier body or a slimmer waistline. You will then have to bear the financial burden of ill health. That's many times more costly than the expense of purchasing and consuming quality food supplements.

So how can you identify quality organically grown whole food nutritional supplements and why won't regular vitamins bought at the local discount store do the same thing? Let's explore that question.

Understanding Nutritional Supplements

If you can't buy organic vegetables, and can't grow them yourself, then whole food nutritional supplements are a viable option.

By taking food supplements, all the work involved with growing organic foods is taken care of for you. It's important to get organically grown foods (or supplements in this case) because most of our country's soil has been depleted of minerals for many decades. Organic farms put a lot of effort into assuring those minerals are in the soil to make them available to the plants as they grow.

Even with an excellent source of quality foods, you should still consider taking quality nutritional supplementation, for a while at least. Why? One reason for supplementation is you cannot change your eating habits quickly enough and you will not be eating enough raw vegetables to get all the phytonutrients, enzymes, and other nutrients your body will need throughout the day. It takes a long time to truly begin eating what you should every day. Food supplements will help you bridge that gap until your eating habits catch up to your daily biological needs.

Plus, you often cannot guarantee the foods you consume have every mineral and enzyme in them you need every day, even if they are organically grown. Nutritional supplements help assure the best and most rounded diet you can get.

Here is a reality check.

You will not appreciate the value and flavor of healthier foods for a considerable length of time. That is why I keep admonishing you that this series of books I am writing are not "diet" books simply to lose weight or achieve some other lofty goal. You've probably tried those in a fit of short-lived enthusiastic exuberance and found them lacking. Rather, this book series espouses lifelong changes in your eating habits using a system to make those changes as easy as possible for you to institute. The goal being to make you healthier and slimmer while enjoying good quality foods.

Changing the eating habits you have indulged in for years or decades will take time and effort. Meanwhile, take organically grown whole food nutritional supplements to bridge the gap. It will make life much easier and better for you.

Whole food nutritional supplements help your gut to heal when Leaky Gut Syndrome is a factor (and it often is). Years of eating poor quality food, processed food, and fatty foods have reduced the ability of your gut to do its job. Such a damaged gut will not efficiently absorb the nutrients you consume.

Nutritional support will help heal your gut tissues so they can become more efficient at absorbing the vitamins and minerals you consume. Unhealthy gut tissues will just let valuable nutrients pass without being absorbed. Then they will be excreted and forever lost to your body. The extra nutrition will also help to make up for some of the nutritional deficiencies resulting from your damaged gut.

Nutritional supplementation is the only way to heal Leaky Gut Syndrome, in addition to changing the consumption of things that caused the condition. There is no magic pill available to reverse the degradation of your gut. Only by eating quality nutrition and food will you be able to give the gut tissues the nutritional building blocks it needs to heal.

Besides, there is only so much food you can consume in one sitting or in one day. Whole food nutritional supplements contain an immense pile of organically grown foods but come in a small package you can easily fit into your belly.

To make these types of supplements, organic foods are ground up and then the water and fiber are removed. All that is left is a concentrated food source. The concentrated food source found in whole food nutritional supplements allow you to consume all the nutrients you need to heal and maintain your body. You could never eat the enormous pile of raw food that is contained in just a few tablets or capsules of a quality nutritional supplement. Having it all in such a small package helps supply these necessary nutrients in a form you can easily consume in one sitting.

You cannot physically eat enough food to get the levels that are recommended for some nutrients. For example, you would have to eat twenty-eight cups of peanuts, five pounds of wheat germ, eight cups of almonds, or drink two quarts of corn oil to get just four hundred international units of vitamin E. It's easier and more practical to take a quality, prepared capsule.

You need a concentrated food source to heal the long-standing nutritional deficiencies you developed over the years while your diet was vastly deficient. You need whole food nutritional supplements, or you will never catch up. If you've never heard of this before, it's not surprising.

It's only when a nutritional deficiency has been longstanding and severe that it presents in clinical ways. You don't know you have nutritional deficiencies until your health fails, and then you never suspect it is due to not having specific nutrients in your daily diet. Most people go to their medical doctor and get a fistful of pills for whatever horrible symptoms they are suffering from, never suspecting a nutritional deficiency is causing their misery.

The programs I organized and outlined in The Lose Weight and Regain Health Series uses proven techniques and methods for improving your health. Usually, these techniques are used by healthcare providers other than medical doctors, though many progressive medical doctors are now using these also... to the significant benefit of their patients. So, if you have only been going to medical doctors for your healthcare, you may have missed out on the most exciting and fastest growing fields in healthcare currently available.

If medical science could not cure you of your health problems, these techniques may give you what you have so desperately been seeking.

And you must ask yourself, "Why haven't I looked at other avenues of healthcare when what I've been doing hasn't been working?"

People with nutritional deficiencies not only have to consume enough quality food to meet their current needs but must make up for nutritional deficiencies that occurred in the past. It's time to play catch-up!

Now that you know you probably have a nutritional deficiency, what can you do about it? Well, take whole food nutritional supplements because your body can produce some vitamins, but it cannot produce minerals.

The only way to be sure you are getting minerals is to eat plants that have been grown in soil containing ample quantities of minerals. These must be the type of plants that can absorb those minerals from the soil and store them in their tissues because not all plants take up all minerals. Also, all soils do not contain every one of the essential minerals your body may need. The soil in specific areas of the country may contain certain minerals while others are totally devoid of them.

Only certain plants will absorb specific minerals and the manufacturers of quality nutritional supplements know which plants can absorb and store them. They grow and use those plants in their products when they want to include those particular minerals in a specific nutritional supplement. To ensure the minerals are present in sufficient quantities for the plants to absorb, the soil is tested and amended regularly.

The conscientious manufacturers of whole food nutritional supplements know all of this and take the time and effort to assay the plant material to make sure enough of the desired mineral is in the plant tissues before they make them into supplements. Then the top-notch manufacturers have biochemists and nutritionists on staff to assay the nutrient and mineral levels in the finished product to assure it has what they think they have in them.

Does that make sense? It makes a lot of sense.

You don't know if the vegetables you buy in the supermarket were grown in soil that contains the minerals you need (they probably weren't) and you don't know if the vegetable you are eating is the type of plant that takes up those particular minerals. There is just no way for you to know these things, so you may easily miss out on getting the minerals you need even when you are trying to eat healthy foods.

It's much simpler to allow the biochemists and nutritionists who make whole food nutritional supplements to formulate supplements that contain everything you need. These professionals make sure the soil has the minerals and nutrients in it, they grow the proper plants to absorb and store those nutrients, and then they test the supplements after they are made to assure all the good stuff is in the supplement. That takes a lot of worry off your mind and is why quality nutritional supplements are not cheap. But they are worth every cent when they keep you from falling into ill health.

All of this is done before they ship the supplements to you. This way, everything is taken care of for you with no effort on your part. Keeping life simple is good!

This is especially true in today's world of depleted soil and polluted environment.

In 1948, spinach held 158 milligrams of iron. Today, raw spinach contains only 27 milligrams of iron. The soil has been depleted of minerals on most of the farms and needs special attention to restore the bioavailability of minerals to the plants.

Not convinced yet? Well, an article from Life Extension Magazine states the quantity of vitamin C in sweet peppers dropped from 128 mg. in 1963 to only 89 mg. in 1975. During this same period, the vitamin A in collard greens dropped from 6,500 I.U. to 3,800 I.U. That's sad and scary at the same time because the people who do not know about this are eating vegetables thinking they're getting all the good stuff their body needs, but that is not true in today's world. It is up to you to find ways around this dire situation, so you and your loved ones do not fall prey to the reality of our modern world and end up trapped in an unhealthy body.

Even when you purchase good produce having an ample supply of minerals, they must be consumed raw otherwise they will lose most of the nutrients in the cooking process. Heat destroys all the enzymes, up to fifty percent of the vitamins, and many of the minerals.

You must eat raw vegetables to avoid destroying these valuable nutrients. However, reality dictates that you are used to eating cooked vegetables and you will continue cooking your vegetables. To work around that, you will need whole food nutritional supplements to make up the difference in lost nutrients until you eat most of your vegetables without cooking them.

Whole food nutritional supplements should be manufactured with a cold pressed process that preserves the vitamins, minerals, and enzymes. Such supplements will have a shelf life listed on the bottle.

You must realize that your body uses these nutritional components in the day-to-day operation of your body, so you must take some every day. Only after today's biological needs are attended to will your body attempt to reverse the deficiencies that have been occurring for most of your life. That's when true healing takes time. It may take months, or even years, for this process to catch up.

It's truly difficult for Americans to grasp this concept because they taught you to think in terms of "healthy" meaning the lack of symptoms and "illness" only existing when you are feeling poorly. Being truly healthy is when all your organs and bodily systems are functioning at one hundred percent efficiency all the time, and that's something you have no way of gauging.

To summarize, you must make up for years of nutritional deficiencies caused by your diet and lifestyle, the way you cook all your food, toxins and other biological stressors, and the lack of nutrients in the soil and, subsequently, your food. With all that going on, I hope you can find some patience to allow your body enough time to catch up and heal.

Chapter 9

Whole Food vs. Fractionalized Molecules

Whole food nutritional supplements have actual food as their source for vital minerals, enzymes, phytonutrients, and vitamins and are not chemicals manufactured in a laboratory. They also have these nutrients in sufficient quantities to make up for any nutritional deficits you may have. "Vitamins" bought at your local discount store probably do not have all these essential nutrients in them… and not in the form in which they occur in nature.

Only nine percent of the American people eat the recommended five servings of fruits and vegetables per day, so it's obvious that as a nation Americans are not very health conscious. If people will not eat nutritional foods, especially raw vegetables and fresh fruit, maybe they will take whole food supplements to stay healthier.

Whole food nutritional supplements contain the whole molecules, just like you find them in the plant that made them. The way they are found in nature, not as they come out of some laboratory somewhere. Manufactured vitamins rarely, if ever, have whole molecules, as they are found in nature. We know these incomplete particles as fractionalized molecules because they are only a portion of the whole molecules whence they came.

It's your choice whether you want whole natural molecules or parts of manufactured molecules. However, you must realize there are several problems with fractionalized molecules. These fractions of molecules must molecularly make themselves whole. It's the nature of molecules.

When you consume a fractionalized molecule, it will steal nutrients from your body to make itself whole. That's not a problem if the newly made whole molecule is not past the portion of the gut tube that can absorb it. The entire gut tube does not absorb all nutrients all the time, and this can cause problems when fractionalized molecules are involved.

There may only be a one-foot section of gut capable of absorbing certain nutrients. If a fractionalized molecule, by the time it steals enough nutrients from your body to make itself whole so your body can absorb it is past the section of gut capable of absorbing it then you lose those nutrients. And that includes the nutrients the fractionalized molecule stole from your body! You end up with less than you had before you consumed the fractionalized molecule. Oops!

You thought you were taking vitamins to be healthier and now you end up losing nutrients in the long run because of the fractionalized molecules found in the manufactured nutrition you consumed. All because you didn't know the difference between whole food nutritional supplements and fractionalized manufactured supplements. Unfortunately, by taking manufactured supplements, you may speed up your descent into ill health and your untimely demise.

Your body is seeking nutrients as they occur in nature, so give it to them in that form. If you can't or won't eat enough raw vegetables and fresh fruit to supply your body with those necessary nutrients, then you should consume whole food nutritional supplements because they are the closest you can get to the way nutrients occur in nature.

A tiny quantity of a vitamin or mineral in its whole food configuration is much more nutritionally effective than fractionalized molecules because it more efficiently satisfies the body's needs. Even if a fractionalized form is taken in larger amounts, it is not as effective, so consume the good stuff and let nature take care of the rest. That way, you do not have to worry about how many milligrams or international units of a vitamin or mineral those supplements contain.

This happens because of the ability of the body to absorb whole food molecules as they occur in plants. Our body recognizes molecules as they occur in nature and readily absorb them. That's simple enough to understand, and it makes sense, doesn't it?

That's why consuming the entire plant, or in this case, the whole food supplement derived from the entire plant, works best. Also, whole food nutritional supplements naturally contain chemical co-factors from the plant used to make them. Many of these co-factors from the plant remain unidentified, but they work together with various nutrients because they have grown together inside the same plant. These co-factors are very important but are absent in manufactured vitamins.

Nutrients and co-factors are naturally balanced inside the plant, and this is how your body is designed to use them. It is this combination of co-factors combined with the naturally occurring vitamins and minerals found along with them in the plant they used to derive whole food nutritional supplements from that is important.

Hopefully, you see that the old saying you can get all the nutrients you need from the food you normally eat regardless of what those foods are is a fallacy. It is a dangerous myth as it makes up a serious threat to the health of you and your family. In other words, you've been lied to. Learn from what we've just reviewed and correct your eating habits to keep yourself and your loved ones healthy.

Understanding Whole Grains

It doesn't matter what your blood type is, there are always some foods in each of the major categories, and that includes grains. This is another group of foods that are often misunderstood, so we will take a few moments to review some of the important facts you need to know.

While the allowed grains vary from one blood type to the next, and your food sensitivity test may show up a few of them to avoid, the fact remains that you may need to learn about a few of the grains you may not be familiar with especially if they are on your highly beneficial foods list when you read about the Eat Right 4 Your Type diet.

Overall, whole grains are good for us, or so it would appear. They make up much of the Mediterranean Diet, which is touted as being good for keeping people healthy and reducing heart and arterial disease. Since the Mediterranean Diet contains many foods that are not only good for people but are easy to use in a variety of recipes, I wrote a book entitled *Modified Mediterranean Diet: Your Bridge to a Slimmer, Healthier Body That Looks and Feels Younger*. This book gives a lot of background on healthy eating but also includes sections on how you can change your favorite recipes to make them into more healthy meal choices you are familiar with and happy to eat.

Whole grains are crucial because they contain more nutrients than refined grains. Why's that important? Because when your body has what it needs nutritionally, your food cravings plunge, and binge eating becomes a thing of the past. It only makes sense to eat nutritionally wholesome foods.

Note that most of what we have been talking about has the word "whole" in it. Whole food nutritional supplements. Whole grains. There's a good reason for that. These are foods as they occur in nature, and your body demands food and the nutrients they contain as nature has provided them. It's the natural way of things. Please don't accept things that are unnatural just because they are more convenient or less expensive. The results are rarely, if ever, good.

But exactly what are whole grains?

In a nutshell, whole grains are grains served in their natural state just as they grow in the fields. Nothing is removed. It's amazing that consumers who recognize the health benefits of whole grains are not entirely sure exactly where to find or how to prepare them for eating.

It is not surprising to find consumers having trouble locating, let alone using, whole grains. While nutritionists suggest that half of your grain consumption be whole grains, whole grains make up only ten to fifteen percent of grain products stocked on supermarket shelves. Whole grains are truly lost amongst the multitudes of refined grain products.

The average American eats less than one serving of whole grains per day. Thirty percent of Americans NEVER eat whole grains. Yet the Department of Health and Human Services, The American Heart Association, and the Healthy People 2010 organization all urge people to eat three to five servings of whole grains per day. The healthful message about whole grains is being lost somewhere along the line.

What comprises a serving of whole grains? A serving is equal to an "ounce-equivalent." That doesn't help much until we put it into layperson's terms we can all understand, right?

A slice of bread or serving of breakfast cereal is considered equal to an ounce. So, three slices of whole grain bread per day satisfy the quantities suggested by these organizations. It's certainly not too difficult to get three slices of bread into yourself every day, is it?

Whole grains are definitely NOT the pasta, cereal, and white bread most folks want to pretend they are.

I don't know how many times I've heard people, in all honesty, say they are eating well because they ate pancakes for breakfast, a pasta salad for lunch, and are planning to have spaghetti for dinner. These misinformed people think that since wheat is a grain, it is fulfilling their daily whole grain requirements.

Trying to explain the difference between refined grains and whole grains to such people only begets a blank stare. They do not, or will not, acknowledge that refined wheat products are not whole grains.

Up to this point, the government has done a very poor job of explaining to the public what a whole grain is, and just as importantly, what it isn't. Let's take a quick lesson at whole grains so you do not make this common mistake.

Whole grain means exactly that. The whole, entire grain as it grows in the field is used as food. Refined grains like the white flour you buy in the supermarket have the fibrous outer shell and other important parts removed during processing.

A lot of fiber, minerals, and vitamins are found in whole grains when compared to their refined brethren.

Antioxidants, including lignans, phenolic acids, and other phytochemicals, are found in whole grains but are removed from refined grain products. These antioxidants may be involved with reducing the risk of heart disease, cancer, and diabetes, so they are important. You should not neglect them.

The Whole Grains Council offers the following definition of exactly what a whole grain is:

"Whole grains or foods made from them contain all the essential parts and naturally occurring nutrients of the entire grain seed. If the grain has been processed (e.g., cracked, crushed, rolled, extruded, and/or cooked), the food product should deliver approximately the same high balance of nutrients that are found in the original grain seed."

Examples of accepted whole grain foods and flours include amaranth, barley, brown and colored rice, buckwheat, bulgur, corn and whole cornmeal, emmer (emmer is known as farro in Italy where it is becoming a very popular food product), millet, oatmeal and whole oats, popcorn, quinoa, sorghum, spelt, teff, triticale, whole rye, whole or cracked wheat, wheat berries, and wild rice.

The sad part is many folks want to eat whole grains but are misled by food suppliers. People eat brown colored bread thinking they make it from whole grains. That's not necessarily the case. You must read the label to determine if the bread truly contains whole grains or is only colored brown for eye appeal.

To make sure you are getting whole grains, you must check the package label. Look for terms such as "Good source of whole grain", "Excellent source of whole grain", or "100% whole wheat."

Beware of food producers that print "whole grain" on the label, while the product contains only a small amount of actual whole grains. Check the ingredient list for terms such as "whole wheat" or "whole oats" listed as the first ingredient. Such products are usually made mostly of whole grains.

If the second ingredient listed is "whole wheat" or "whole oats" it may have as little as one percent of these grains or as much as forty-nine percent. Stick with products listing some type of whole grain as the first ingredient.

The term "multi-grain" is useless in determining how much of the product truly contains whole grains. Do not be misled by this term unless the first ingredient is listed as being a whole grain.

The best way to determine if a food product has whole grains in sufficient quantities is to look for the Whole Grain Stamp. Actually, there are three Whole Grain Stamps. Each signifies a differing quantity of whole grains in that product.

The first whole grain stamp shows the product in question contains a half serving of whole grain, while the second stamp means it has a full serving of whole grain. The third stamp specifies that all the grains in that product are whole grains.

When the Whole Grain Stamp is on the food packaging, you don't have to worry about reading the ingredients list if you are concerned about how much whole grains are contained in that product. That can save you some time, so begin looking for it on the whole grain products you buy.

A good example of "truth in advertising" comes from the Whole Grain Council. You can visit the Council's website and visit the web page listing food producers and products using the Whole Grain Stamp. The information on the Whole Grains Council website offers an easy way to find whole grain foods that are pre-made, convenient to buy, and consume.

Since whole grains have traditionally been available in their natural state, and mostly sold only in health food stores, it has created problems for the typical American consumer. Most consumers have not taken the time to learn how to cook or develop a taste for these healthy grains.

By perusing the products listed at the Whole Grain Council's site, you can locate foods ranging from sliced bread to lasagna noodles that are excellent sources of whole grains. Readily available pre-made whole grain products expand the potential for utilizing whole grains in your favorite recipes.

It is felt that less refined foods like whole grains (and other foods such as legumes, which are not being specifically discussed) slow down the absorption rate of food. Slower absorption rates help prevent sharp spikes in insulin secretion, which puts less stress on your body.

In theory at least, this should help reduce the incidence of problems like diabetes. In fact, that is exactly what was found by several studies. The more whole grain and fiber people consumed resulted in fewer instances of diabetes occurring when compared to a diet higher in refined carbohydrates like potatoes, white bread, and refined grain pasta.

Researchers at Tufts University found that people eating three or more servings of whole grains per day are less likely to develop insulin resistance and metabolic syndrome. They found that high fiber cereals were especially good at preventing these types of problems.

Think of dietary fiber in your gut as being a slurry of material. I always visualize a slurry as being like liquid concrete being poured. If you haven't seen concrete being poured at a construction site, think of a thick milkshake with chunks of fruit, like strawberry or peach, floating around in it. That's a slurry.

Nutrients, as well as fats and sugars, are only absorbed when they contact the gut wall. Not while they're tumbling around in the middle of the slurry. The fibrous slurry (officially called chyme) stops nutrients from being absorbed all at one time. Only when the nutrients emerge from the center of the slurry and rub up against the gut wall can they be absorbed, slowing the absorption process.

The slower absorption of fats and sugars results in reducing the amount of cholesterol and sugar in the bloodstream. Slower absorption of these nutrients is illustrative of one aspect of how dietary fiber may aid people who suffer from high cholesterol or diabetes.

Similar research findings occurred when scientists studied heart disease and its relationship to dietary fiber. Interestingly, test subjects with higher dietary fiber consumption derived from whole grains had a lower risk of heart disease than those whose dietary fiber came from fruit and vegetables.

Are vegetables and fruit important? They are, but so are whole grains. Make sure you include them in your daily diet.

Researchers in the U.S. as well as in Europe found that for each ten grams of fiber consumed per day, there was a fourteen percent lower risk of having a heart attack. When a heart attack occurred, there was a twenty-five percent lower risk of dying from it.

A group of researchers from the Harvard School of Public Health showed that study participants eating over forty grams of fiber per day cut their chance of having a heart attack by almost twenty percent. So, including fiber in your diet sounds like a good way to hedge your bet of avoiding or surviving a heart attack.

But why does eating whole grains offer protection from heart attack?

Researchers at the Jean Mayer USDA Human Nutrition Research Center on Aging at Tufts University found that eating six servings of whole grains or more per week resulted in a slower build-up of plaque in the arteries. Some researchers speculate high antioxidant levels in whole grains may be why a slower accumulation of plaque occurs.

Whole grains contain antioxidants equaling or exceeding the amounts found in fruit and vegetables. For example, corn has almost twice the antioxidant content of apples. They found wheat and oats to have almost the same quantity of antioxidants as broccoli and spinach. That's good to remember because whole grains are more palatable to some people than are vegetables and fruit, so they may be more inclined to consume it, even though it is best to eat them all.

Just remember, we are discussing whole grain corn, wheat, and oats. If the corn is degerminated or the wheat is refined, the antioxidant advantage is lost.

Studies continue surfacing, showing that free radicals are formed in the bloodstream as sugar consumption increases (or things easily converted to sugar such as refined carbohydrates). They particularly found this in people having an unhealthy accumulation of body fat, which is most Americans.

Free radicals attack the walls of arteries and cause damage. Arterial damage caused by free radicals appears as little holes in the walls of the artery, and that's not a good thing. The body must continually repair the arterial damage by plugging the holes with cholesterol.

Just like "The Little Dutch Boy" who saved his village from flooding by plugging the hole in the dike with his finger, cholesterol plugs keep the blood inside the blood vessels where it belongs. However, the continual damage incurred by people who constantly eat foods leading to a rise in blood sugar demands the body repair the damage to the blood vessels with cholesterol plugs. Continual repair with cholesterol results in a build-up of plaque in the artery.

Voila! Cholesterol plaque forms, and these people are on their way to a heart attack or stroke.

They usually blame cholesterol for clogged arteries when it is really sugar consumption and an unhealthy accumulation of body fat that may be the more likely precipitating factor leading to a heart attack or stroke. The antioxidants of whole grain foods stop the actions of the free radicals, thereby reducing or stopping damage to the arteries. Lack of arterial damage means there is no need for the body to repair the blood vessels with cholesterol. The result is arteries free of plaque (or at least reduced plaquing) and the frequency of heart attack or stroke is greatly reduced.

However, don't be fooled into thinking eating fiber by itself can achieve the same results as eating whole grains. All too often, people swap the terms fiber and whole grains like they are the same thing, but they are not interchangeable. Fiber is usually found in whole grains, but whole grains contain many other beneficial components.

In our fast-paced world, everyone wants things faster and easier. Food choices are not exempt from this desire. Witness the rise in the popularity of fast foods.

When fiber was administered in capsule form, it was not nearly as effective as when whole grains were consumed. Easier to eat? Yes. But better? No.

All the other "stuff" found in whole grains is very important. Things like antioxidants, copper, magnesium, phenolic acids, phytic acid, and selenium are found in whole grains but not necessarily in fiber alone.

It is not just the presence of these other factors that make whole grains more effective in reducing the incidence of heart disease. The fact they act synergistically with each other to perform their varied tasks is significant.

Unfortunately, the scientific community has not yet figured out the exact synergistic relationship of these factors to each other. That's OK though, we only need to understand that we need to eat whole grains to assure we get all the good "stuff" working together for our benefit. Give the scientists time to do their work while we enjoy the benefits of whole grains.

They linked some cancers to the absence of adequate fiber in the diet. This is especially true when the fiber should come from whole grains, fresh fruits, and raw vegetables. The most promising research appears to point toward a cancer prevention diet being rich in fiber from whole grains, fresh fruits, and raw vegetables while being low in fat. Once again, the combination of all the "good stuff" as found naturally in whole grains, fruits, and vegetables seems to be the key.

Eventually, scientists may figure out the intricate interactions involved amongst these various food nutrients in preventing disease. Until then, just eat the good stuff the way nature and God intended.

Don't try reducing everything down to the least common denominator to simplify things. All the food components may have to work in harmony with each other. The interplay of nature's nutrients working together for your benefit may be the key.

Besides the antioxidants found in whole grains, the bulkiness of dietary fiber reduces the time food spends in the gut tube. The faster waste products are expelled from the body, the less time toxins in the waste have to act upon the bowel walls. Reduced waste exposure time is important to prevent the formation of serious conditions such as cancer of the bowel. It is much easier to reduce the incidence of bowel cancers by eating more dietary fiber than attempting to cure it after it becomes a life-threatening problem.

A team of researchers at the University of Utah found that eating vegetables, fruits, and whole grains reduced the risk of rectal cancer by twenty-seven to thirty-one percent. For people eating over thirty-four grams of fiber per day, it reduced the risk of rectal cancer by sixty-six percent. That seems to show that the more dietary fiber you consume from raw vegetables, fresh fruits, and whole grains, the less chance you have of developing rectal cancer. Eat the good stuff and you may never know how many bad things you avoided.

Keep waste moving through your body quickly and efficiently. That's the way things are supposed to work. To put off the act of elimination because you are "too busy" is foolhardy. When the "call of nature" yells at you, answer it! Eating foods such as whole grains along with a lot of water will keep things moving through you the way they are supposed to.

Because of the bulky nature of dietary fiber in the gut, it is important to drink plenty of water. And I mean PLENTY of water. Most of the bulk found in fiber is because of the high water content. If water is not present in sufficient quantities to keep the fiber soft, you will feel you are passing a brick on your next trip to the bathroom. Try to avoid that unpleasant situation by drinking a lot of water throughout each day.

Preventing disease is nice, but how does eating whole grains help with an unhealthy accumulation of body fat? That's a good question since an unhealthy accumulation of body fat seems to be intimately related to many of the disease processes we have been discussing.

A review of the health records of 72,000 men found those eating at least forty grams of whole grains per day could cut middle-age weight gain by up to 3.5 pounds. To put this into perspective, just one cup of oatmeal or two slices of whole-wheat bread provides at least forty grams of whole grain nutrition per day.

In a similarly sized study, researchers at the Harvard School of Public Health tracked over 74,000 women and found that the women getting a greater percentage of their total food intake from whole grains weighed less on average than those who ate fewer whole grains.

But exactly how much is forty grams of whole grains? Do you have any idea? Let's take a minute to study this.

A serving of whole grains in 100% whole wheat bread is sixteen grams. So, doing the math, we see that 2.5 slices of whole wheat bread roughly equals forty grams of whole grains. It's not a lot of food, so you should be able to fit it into your daily diet with no problems.

Changing your whole grain eating habits to include at least forty grams of whole grains every day can reap tremendous health benefits while keeping you slimmer. Remember what I said about getting healthier to become slimmer?

How many grams are found in a 100% whole grain English muffin? One half of the muffin will give you about sixteen grams. As will two cups of popped popcorn or one-third cup of cooked whole wheat pasta. That's not an enormous pile of food, is it? Luckily, whole grains fill you up quickly, especially if you drink the required amount of water with them.

Food manufacturers jumped on the "Low fat" and "Fat-free" craze and just about killed everyone. When the fat was taken out, immense quantities of sugars were added to give the products some flavor, and consumers ended up eating much more of these foods.

There are two suspected reasons consumers ate greater quantities of low fat and fat-free products. Consumers either didn't feel fulfilled eating these foods or they thought it was OK to eat more because the foods didn't have fat and were, therefore, healthy.

This resulted in consumers getting fatter with their arteries clogging faster due to sugar-induced plaque formation. So much for another supposedly good idea popularized by the media.

If there is a demand for whole grain foods in the ready-to-eat form, the producers will supply such foods in no time flat. Capitalism is a great thing when there is a demand to be satisfied.

Up to this point, there has not been an enormous demand for whole grain products, though the demand is growing as the health benefits and great taste of whole grains become better known. The number of whole grain products on supermarket shelves is slowly increasing all the time.

Recently, there have been several new products containing whole grains introduced to the marketplace. Most are quite tasty and are not radically different from their refined grain counterparts. This will make your transition to increasing your whole grain consumption much easier.

In the bigger scheme of things, if food manufacturers began producing true whole grain products, the demand for whole grains would increase tremendously. In a small way, this is already occurring.

Such a situation may benefit the family farmers who are working with sub-optimal lands. The small farmer is having trouble competing in world markets by growing the currently popular crops. Small farming operations may increase their profit margins by growing whole grains. Competing on the world market with corn and soybeans may not be as profitable as switching to other grain products.

Biodiversity in our food supply is a good thing. If the demand for whole grains increased from the current ten to fifteen percent of total grain foods currently found on supermarket shelves, everyone from the farmer to the consumer would benefit. Especially when you eat whole grains and reap the health benefits they offer.

Chapter 11

Learning to Eat More Whole Grains

You may have an aversion to certain foods and it's likely because of what you learned to eat when you were a small child. To put this discussion on learning how to eat more whole grains, let's look at how you can train your children to like the foods that are going to make them healthier. It will be eating habits they can carry on throughout their entire lifespan so they can continue enjoying improved health. It's one of the best gifts you can give your kids. The same principles apply to you, so just because we will discuss children, you can use the same techniques to change your eating habits.

Here we go.

Your kids probably eat junk because it's what you taught them to eat. Baby birds eat worms because mom and dad bird taught them to eat worms. Your kids eat soda and fat laden snacks because you taught them to eat junk food.

What if you were to teach your children to eat whole grains, raw vegetables, and fresh fruit?

It can be done, it truly can. All it takes is concerted and systematic efforts on your part to not only supply these types of foods, but to eat them yourselves. It just won't work if your kids have raw carrots and celery sticks to snack on while you stuff your face with potato chips. They watch you and learn from you in all aspects of life, and that includes their eating habits.

If you're serious about changing your family's diet and the kids are too old to change their eating habits overnight, whole grains are the place to begin. Begin replacing your usual white bread with a whole wheat or whole oat product over the next three weeks by keeping both types of bread in your house. After the three weeks are up, just stop buying the white bread.

If the "good stuff" is the only bread available, they will begin eating it. If not, they won't starve. Believe me. Kids won't starve if food is available. However, if junk food is available with the healthy stuff, they will gorge themselves on the junk. It's what you taught them and it's most likely what you were taught as well.

Which is why you must begin replacing junk food with raw vegetables and fresh fruit. It will amaze you at how quickly kids will go to the refrigerator for a ready-to-eat carrot stick if potato chips are not available.

Raw vegetables and fruit may be foreign to your taste buds and you may be reluctant to eat them. Interestingly, after eating them for a while, you will be surprised that a vegetable can be so tasty eaten raw.

Yes, even a little tidbit like cauliflower. It's a neglected vegetable many people would have never dreamed of trying to eat without being cooked until mushy then smothered in cheese or butter. It has a distinctive and pleasing flavor all its own if you give it a chance. The flavor has been described as "peppery" or "spicy." You will never experience the awakening of your taste buds until you eat it raw.

It may be hard to believe, but eating raw vegetables will have an allure all by itself once you can appreciate their intrinsic taste and texture. At that point, you will begin to fully appreciate the subtle flavors.

Switch to fruit and vegetables as you replace white bread with whole grain varieties. And I mean varieties. Rotating between three or four different breads makes it easier for the kids to choose what they want. It keeps things from getting boring for them. Eventually, they will begin preferring one type or brand of whole grain bread over the others. That simplifies your buying decisions and the kid's transition to whole grains has taken an astronomical leap forward. Yes, it becomes cumbersome to have three different breads available at the same time, but everyone can find something to suit his or her taste. Everyone loves variety, at least until they form a preference for one whole grain bread over the others.

As you are transitioning to whole grains, fruits, and vegetables, don't forget you have to add some healthy foods into your meal planning. Add a salad as the first course at a dinner that includes a bit of whole grain. Add a whole grain as a side dish along with the mashed potatoes. Ultimately, you will slowly begin leaving the mashed potatoes off the menu and serve only the whole grain side dish.

Nothing says you must go "cold turkey" changing your long-established eating habits. Just remember to set a deadline when you want to have the transition to healthy eating accomplished. Give yourself plenty of time and be realistic about your goals. Slowly adding new foods to your meal planning and deleting those that are not so healthy will take weeks or even months. Don't rush it or you will meet tremendous resistance from everyone in the family.

It will surprise you how quickly the transition to healthier foods will occur if you don't buy junk food on one food-shopping trip. This will give everyone time to clean up the junk food in your house. Then on the next trip you only buy one, repeat, ONE bag of junk snacks and ONE bottle of soda. On your third trip to the supermarket, you will still buy one bag of snacks and one bottle of soda.

Just remember to have the good stuff available from the beginning. Fruit juice will soon replace soda as a staple in your diet. Whole grains will sneak easily onto your plate at dinner. Whole wheat and whole oat bread will grace your lunch sandwich. Fresh fruit will replace the snack cake in the lunch boxes and a whole grain cereal will have long ago replaced the sugar-laden horror for breakfast.

Eventually, only fresh fruit, vegetables, and whole grains will find their way into your shopping cart. The trip to the supermarket goes much faster when you don't go down the junk food aisles.

Most lifestyle and eating changes are doomed to failure because everyone is terribly enthusiastic at the beginning. Maybe you made a New Year's Resolution or are determined to lose weight by summer and take up the healthy lifestyle of your favorite movie star.

You may try to eat all raw vegetables or fresh fruit while forsaking all the foods you were raised with. This effort will only last a very short time before you fall back into your old eating habits and then you will feel like a failure. You don't need demolished self-esteem complicating your transition into healthier eating habits.

Take your time. By adding more whole grains, vegetables, and fruits to your regular diet, you will live longer so you will have more time to make more changes. Slow but sure is the way to change you and your family's eating habits.

It won't take long before you notice an interesting change in eating behaviors. You will note everyone is choosing healthier foods even when unhealthy choices are available. Believe me, it will happen if you are diligent and determined.

So, until the food suppliers catch up to you and begin producing the ready-to-eat whole grain foods you want, what do you do? Well, you must buy those that are available and learn a little about whole grains and how to prepare them. Let's investigate that now.

Chapter 12

Whole Grain Primer

There are several whole grains available and they differ considerably, so you should have a fun time experimenting with them all. Some are easier to find in stores than others, but if you shop in the right stores (or look online) you can always find what you are looking for. You will like some of these whole grains immediately and others will not be to your liking. Find those you like and begin using them in your daily food regimen. Let's take a closer look at the available whole grains.

Amaranth

Amaranth is high in quality protein but has no gluten. Therefore, if you want to use it in leavened breads, it must be mixed with wheat flour. Wheat has gluten, which is why it gives foods "good chew," but this form of wheat is usually a refined grain and is not a whole grain with all the benefits we discussed. When I try to define what "good chew" is, I imagine pizza dough. The "chew" is often the best part of pizza dough and is what makes pizza such a highly sought-after and fun food to eat.

Amaranth is often used in bread, cereal, pancakes, muffins, and crackers, so there are lots of ways to prepare it.

Barley

Barley has a tough outer hull that is difficult to remove, so a portion of the bran is always lost in processing. Lightly pearled barley is not technically a whole grain as some of the bran is missing but they still considered it to be healthier than refined grains. Barley may lower cholesterol better than oat fiber, which is an impressive and very useful attribute.

Since barley is grown in a variety of climates, it is an adaptable crop beneficial for farmers. If the demand for barley were greater, everyone would benefit.

Buckwheat

Technically, buckwheat is not really a whole grain, and it is not a type of wheat. Then what is it? It is related to rhubarb. Can you see why this business of finding, understanding, and eating whole grains is difficult?

Regardless, buckwheat is so good it has found a home amongst the whole grains. While it is best known as the basis for some fantastic pancakes, it is also used to make soba noodles in Japan, crepes in Britain, and kasha in Russia.

Health wise, they have found buckwheat to contain large quantities of rutin. Rutin has been shown to be good for blood vessels and helps prevent atherosclerotic plaques from forming.

Healthcare practices use nutritional supplements high in rutin to nutritionally support the blood vessels to strengthen them, so people don't bruise easily. If you bruise easily, strongly consider putting buckwheat at the top of your list of whole grains to enjoy regularly.

Buckwheat is a very resilient plant and grows in poor soils, even on rocky hillsides, and doesn't need chemical pesticides to thrive. It's another plant that would be beneficial for farmers in certain areas if it were more popular with the consumer.

Bulgur

Bulgur is the basis of several popular dishes. Both as a main course and as a side dish. Many people also use it as an addition to salads after it is cooked. Obviously, it's a very versatile whole grain that can be used in many tasty dishes.

Bulgur is boiled wheat, which is then dried and finally cracked. Because it has been previously cooked, it only needs to be boiled for ten minutes before being ready to eat. If you need a fast base for a meal, bulgur is a good choice. It is very high in fiber and because of its ease of preparation and mild flavor, is an excellent candidate for your first foray into the world of whole grains.

Because of its mild flavor, it is good to use in place of spaghetti and pastas in your favorite dishes. Don't expect it to be exactly like spaghetti because it won't be. Use it with your favorite recipes, but mentally look upon it as a new dish unto itself, because that is what it will be.

Corn

Almost everyone is familiar with corn in one form or another. The trick is to read the labels to see if the corn has been degerminated. If it has been degerminated, it lacks the germ portion of the grain, so it is no longer considered to be a whole grain.

It is interesting to note that whole grain corn has twice the antioxidant activity of apples, meaning it has more antioxidants than any other grain or vegetable. That's important to remember.

While corn has been berated as a vegetable, it is getting a second look from many health-minded individuals. It is important to realize that when corn is consumed with beans, the protein value increases because it creates a complimentary mix of amino acids. That's good news for us humans!

Emmer (Farro)

Emmer, or as it is known in Italy, Farro, is an ancient strain of wheat. It's been used for so long that the Roman legions ate it as part of their daily rations. Sadly, it is hard to find today because durum wheat, which is much easier to hull, has replaced it.

After being refined, which you do not want because it is no longer a whole grain, emmer is the basis for semolina flour and is considered by some as being the best choice for making refined grain pasta.

In its whole grain form, emmer can be used as a tasty substitute for pasta in your favorite recipes. Its mild flavor allows it to be used in many ways, so don't be afraid to experiment with it.

Grano

Grano is another one of those grains having a tough outer hull that, when removed, results in the loss of some of the bran. Therefore, it may not technically be a whole grain at all, though it is still healthier than fully refined grains.

Grano, wheat berries, and bulgur are all made from the same durum wheat, so let's discuss them together. Because Grano has some of its tough outer hull removed, it cooks faster than wheat berries and is ready to eat after only a half hour of boiling.

Wheat berries are whole wheat kernels that can be used as a side dish or breakfast cereal. However, because their tough outer hull is still in place, they must be boiled for up to an hour (preferably after soaking overnight). That makes wheat berries a little more difficult to use than some of the other whole grains we have been discussing.

Bulgur has already been boiled, and then dried, so it cooks in about 10 minutes. The difference among these three forms of durum wheat is the way they were processed, how much of the original hull and bran remains, and the cooking times. Naturally, the lesser bran of Grano will mediate some of its beneficial effects when compared to the other two whole grain products.

Millet

While millet is a leading food grain used in India, China, Russia, the Himalayas, and South America, here in the United States, it is mainly used for bird feed. It has a very delicate flavor that must be brought out by roasting or by adding it to other dishes.

While listed as a whole grain, millet is actually a seed. It's gluten-free, easily digested, high in fiber, and low on the glycemic index, which may help keep your blood sugar levels stable.

Depending on how it's cooked, millet recipes can have a creamy texture like mashed potatoes or a fluffier consistency like rice. Look on the Internet for millet recipes and it will surprise you how quickly you use it as a basis for many tasty meals.

Oats

Here is one of my personal favorites!

Most often used as a hot breakfast cereal in the United States, it has many uses. Interestingly, oats almost always have all its bran and germ intact as you find it on the store shelf. This is rather unique among the whole grains. It's a comfort knowing you are buying the most beneficial form of the grain. It also retains its bran and germ layer, even when it is ground into flour.

Oats come in several forms. They can be flattened to form rolled oats or steamed and flattened to create "quick oats." The more the oats are processed, the faster they cook.

Personally, I prefer steel-cut oats. They take about forty-five minutes to cook, which is a long time in the morning, but it is worth it. The flavor is much richer than rolled oats and way ahead of "quick oats" in my humble opinion.

Steel-cut oats are also known by the names "Irish" or "Scottish" oats. They are the whole oat grain that has only been cut in half to aid in water penetration, so they will cook faster. If you have been turned off by the bland taste of the quick oats your mother forced you to eat as a child you will really be surprised by the rich, nutty flavor of steel-cut oats. Do yourself a favor and try them.

Oats, like barley, contain a specific type of fiber called Beta-glucan. Beta-glucan has been very effective in lowering cholesterol. Some recent research studies have shown oats may be effective in helping to prevent arterial plaque formation.

Quinoa

Quinoa (pronounced Keen-Wah) is originally from South America. It thrives at high altitude and is a popular crop to grow in the Rocky Mountain area of the United States.

They often use it as a side dish because it is light and fluffy. They also use quinoa in soups, salads, or baked dishes. It is easy to use because it fits busy lifestyles by cooking in ten to twelve minutes.

Quinoa is being used more and more in breakfast cereals and other processed food products. Its major benefit is found in the fact it contains whole proteins. This means all the essential amino acids our body cannot produce on its own are found in quinoa.

This is an important fact for those calling themselves "vegetarians" because they eat only vegetables while avoiding meat, eggs, milk, etc. Being a vegetarian is fine if you do it correctly. Most do not and they pay the price by putting themselves into an unhealthy state. It takes a lot of effort and learning to eat a totally vegetarian diet. Please take the time to read up on the subject and do things correctly if you are so inclined.

Rice

Whole grain rice is usually brown but may be red or black with a mix of hues in between. Brown rice is lower in fiber than most other whole grains.

The white rice most of you are familiar with has been refined and is not considered to be a whole grain. All its bran and germ have been removed, so most of its benefits have been discarded.

They commonly use rice as a baby's first solid food because it is the most easily digested grain. They also report it to be good for folks who are gluten intolerant.

Rye

Rye can grow in areas too cold or wet for other crops. This is another plant worth consideration for farmers with less-than-ideal soil or growing conditions.

Rye is especially useful for diabetics because it has a low glycemic index because of the high fiber content of its bran and endosperm. This is a rather unusual situation in whole grains and makes rye unique.

The type of fiber found in rye makes you feel full quickly, offering an obvious benefit for weight loss.

Sorghum (Milo)

In the United States, sorghum is mostly grown to feed animals or made into wallboard or bio-degradable packing material. If it is made into cardboard, it must be tasty and good for you, right? All joking aside, it is good for you. It is especially useful to those suffering from celiac disease because it does not contain gluten.

Just because we do not use it as a major food item in the United States does not mean it is not tasty. Worldwide, it is an important food crop for humans. This is just another example of Americans not eating what is good for us. This is a shame because sorghum is very drought resistant and can be grown in areas inhospitable to other crops.

Across the globe, sorghum is made into porridge, popped like popcorn, and made into bread or beer. It's truly an interesting and versatile whole grain that deserves more attention from consumers.

Spelt

Spelt is a great grain, in my opinion. I really love its rich, nutty flavor when it's made into bread. Toasted spelt bread, with a smattering of real butter, adds a lot as a side to a hot bowl of soup on a cold winter eve. It doesn't have the high gluten content of our more common refined wheat flours and is therefore crumblier. However, it is still satisfying to chew.

I was pleasantly surprised to see a local bread bakery making a special run of spelt bread every two weeks. You must order your spelt bread ahead of time, but it is worth the wait.

Spelt is reported to have been around since biblical times. It has been reported that some folks who are sensitive to refined wheat can eat spelt. However, there are no reliable studies to prove this, so be careful if you try it.

Teff

Teff grains are tiny. It is usually only found in places like Ethiopia, India, and Australia. In Ethiopia, it is an important food crop made into a type of flatbread.

Teff is a form of millet and is easy to grow. It's very versatile and is often used to make porridge or is added to various baked items. It is always used as a whole grain because it is too small to grind efficiently.

Teff has twice the quantity of iron found in other whole grains and is high in calcium. One cup of cooked teff has more calcium than a cup of milk. That's about twenty times more calcium than other whole grains.

Triticale

The protein found in triticale comes in a form that is easily absorbed by the body and is much more abundant than the proteins found in wheat or soybeans. Triticale is a hybrid of durum wheat and rye that grows without commercial fertilizers or pesticides. That's important, as pesticides are a prime source of xenohormones capable of mimicking estrogen, which can lead to estrogen dominance. Estrogen dominance is to be avoided if you expect to maintain a healthy amount of body fat.

Wheat

Wheat is well known to us as many of our foods are made from it. Wheat's principal claim to fame is that it contains large quantities of gluten, which makes appetizing risen breads and other baked goods. However, this same gluten causes havoc with those suffering from celiac disease.

Wild Rice

Interestingly, wild rice is not rice at all. It is a seed from aquatic grasses. Wild rice has twice the protein and fiber of brown rice. It is expensive, so it is often mixed with other types of rice or grains before being served.

That's all very nice. Now we know what whole grains are, but what do we do with them?

Well, there are always cookbooks showing how to cook whole grains that are available at, or can be ordered from, your local bookseller. You can also look on the Internet for booksellers offering cookbooks. The Internet itself offers free whole grain recipes at various sites. All you need to do is search for "whole grain recipes." Until then, you can just be creative and begin adding whole grains into your usual recipes. Add them in slowly and no one will notice. You may be pleasantly surprised if everyone soon prefers the variety containing whole grains.

Here are a few tips to get you thinking about adding whole grains to your diet. These suggestions can be changed to suit your tastes:

- Substitute half of the white flour in your cookie, bread, muffin, and pancake recipes with whole-wheat flour. If you are adventurous, you can add up to twenty percent of another whole grain, such as sorghum. It's fun and exciting to experiment with less familiar grains.

- Add a half-cup of bulgur, wild rice, oats, or barley to your bread stuffing recipes.

Oats are a great grain to add to many of the recipes you have used for years. For instance, you can add oats to your favorite zucchini bread recipe or substitute oat flour for some of the refined flour called for in a zucchini bread recipe.

It is easy to make oat flour. Just put dry oats in your blender and blend away. It makes quite a tornado of flying oats and becomes usable flour in a short time.

Try "overstuffing" oatmeal cookies by adding extra oats to oatmeal-raisin cookies. They are still cookies and are higher in sugar and calories than you want most of your foods to be, but you must live in the real world. Cookies are important in the real world! Just keep them as healthy as possible.

Adding double the quantity of oats called for in an apple crisp recipe will do the same thing. Check some of your favorite recipes and see where you can make whole grain substitutions or add extra if they are already included in the recipe.

If you were to deny yourselves the sweet, tasty snacks you have become accustomed to, you will soon end up falling back into your old eating habits. That won't help you at all, so go slowly as you experiment, adding whole grains to your favorite recipes.

Adding oats to meatballs and meatloaf works well. No one will complain because the oats are so well hidden. Add an egg or two to hold it all together. It is easy to be creative and add whole grains to many of your favorite recipes.

Add a half-cup of cooked wheat berries, rye berries, wild rice, brown rice, sorghum, or barley to your favorite canned or homemade soups. Just remember to add whole grain products at the time of serving otherwise the grains will soak up most of the liquid. This is especially important when storing soups, as you will end up with a soup without broth. Storing soup and cooked grains separately will avoid this problem. If you want the grains to soak up some of the flavor of the broth, simply make extra broth and cook the grains separately from the soup.

There are many soup recipes in the cookbooks you currently have that will benefit from adding whole grains. Scan your cookbooks and see where you can insert whole grains into those recipes.

With soup, it is usually a good idea to add the cooked whole grains to the bowl first, then add the soup broth. This is an easy way to gauge the quantity of grains you want to eat.

Whole grain corn meal is another easy grain to use to increase your whole grain consumption. Use whole grain corn meal (the type that does not say "degerminated") in corn cakes, corndodgers, corn bread, corn mush (both fresh and fried), corn fritters, corn bread, and corn muffins. These recipes are commonly found in cookbooks you may already have on hand.

Make risottos, pilafs, and other rice type dishes with whole grains like barley, brown rice, bulgur, millet, quinoa, and sorghum. The different tastes are only restricted by your imagination.

A mix of various whole grains sometimes makes a superior recipe compared to the one you have become accustomed to. If you find you have created a new and better recipe, be sure to write it down. You can even go as far as giving it a new name to avoid making comparisons with its parent recipe. The whole grain recipe deserves an opportunity to stand alone.

Many whole grain breads are available in the supermarket. Whole grain breads, including pita bread, are easy to introduce to your family. Many kids prefer whole grain breads to white bread once they became used to them.

For several months, I always had both types of bread on hand for my children's school lunch sandwiches. Soon they began preferring the whole grain varieties. One child likes the multi-grain bread that has whole grains listed first in the ingredient list, while another likes whole grain rye bread. Kids enjoy having choices, so give them a wide range of alternatives.

It's a lot of different types of bread to have in our house but it all is eaten. That's the bottom line.

Another easy way to add whole grains to your recipes is to buy whole grain pastas, or a blend of whole and refined grains. These foods require a new mindset because they are vastly different from refined grain products. That's OK if you know what to expect.

This is one of those instances where you may want to start with your usual recipe, but name the dish something else. It may sound like a stupid idea at first, but it is a psychological technique that will allow you to transition to healthier eating habits. You may even have to change a recipe to make it more palatable to your personal tastes when using whole grain pastas.

For example, if you make a huge batch of "Aunt May's Lasagna" with whole grain lasagna noodles, you will be disappointed. It's not that it will not be a tasty dish, but when you substitute whole grain lasagna noodles for the refined grain noodles Good Old Aunt May used in her recipe, it will totally change the character of the dish.

Your preconceived notion of what Aunt May's lasagna is supposed to taste like will not be met when using whole grain lasagna noodles. So don't try making Aunt May's lasagna with whole grain noodles. Instead, make "Tasty Spelt Noodles with Mushroom Marinara Sauce."

Psychologically, you have just established an association between a great tasting meal and your mental picture of what to expect. It may seem like a silly exercise, but it's important to re-program your idea of what to expect when you make a certain dish.

Look for cereals that are already prepared and ready-to-eat in your supermarket. Both hot and cold cereals made with whole grains like Kamut, kasha, buckwheat, or spelt are readily available in most supermarkets these days.

Many local supermarkets have a portion of the cereal section dedicated to nothing but whole grain cereals. Most of these are very tasty! The food producers have caught on to the fact Americans need some type of sweetener in their cereals or they won't continue buying them. So, the producers are using foods like concentrated cherry juice to sweeten their whole grain cereals. This combination really works and makes a very palatable product.

I like hot cereals in the wintertime, but cold cereals get the nod on busy mornings. My children prefer cold cereals, so we always have a selection of both hot and cold whole grain cereals on hand. Determine what your family prefers by giving them several choices.

I get bored with food quickly. But with cold breakfast cereals, I have found a solution to this problem. To keep things interesting, I mix two different cereals in the same bowl. Sometimes I just add the two together, while at other times I put one cereal on one side of the bowl and another on the other side of the bowl. Besides, by having two different whole grains in one meal, you get the different benefits each offers. This health aspect should not be overlooked.

It's silly, but it maintains variety for me. Besides, it's an easy way to make a single bowl of cold cereal into a two-course meal!

Yeah, I know it's ridiculous, but it works for me. It just may work for you, too. Anything that will be helpful in getting more whole grains into your daily diet is worth a try. Don't be afraid of being creative and experiment.

How important is the addition of whole grains to your diet? According to one study that dealt strictly with the consumption of whole grain and refined grain cereals as it relates to weight gain in men, they found breakfast cereals to be important in weight control. The researchers concluded that consuming cereals, regardless of whether they are whole grains or refined grains, lowers the risk of obesity. Breakfast cereals make up much of our total grain intake. It is suspected that the consumption of whole grain cereals may even be more effective in reducing weight than cereals containing refined grains.

Regardless of how you look at it, whole grains are good for you. Use them to help get your health back, then maintain it.

Chapter 13

Summary

You learned how to establish a symptom survey, measure body parts, and then use that information to monitor your body's reaction to the changes you make in your diet. When a symptom disappears or at least reduces in intensity after you institute dietary changes, it becomes one of your canaries. Your canaries are what you will monitor weekly to make sure you are not allowing foods that are harmful to you to slip back into your diet.

You also learned that you must read Eat Right 4 Your Type by Dr. Peter J. D'Adamo to find out which foods are beneficial to you, which ones are neutral, and which ones to avoid as though they are poison. After you established the dietary changes outlined in that book, you learned how to use food sensitivity tests to fine-tune the foods you should be avoiding.

We looked at the intelligence of consuming organically grown vegetables and covered whole grains and ways you can increase the consumption of these beneficial foods.

If you want to maximize your health to its fullest extent, you can read the *Executive Summary and Workbook* which includes all steps I outline to discover how to fine tune your diet so you can discover the foods your body wants and which ones it does not want. Each step in the process takes you deeper into discovering the foods you must avoid based on your unique individual needs.

The *Executive Summary and Workbook* includes not only the information found in this book but also the rest of the steps to fine tune your eating habits as found in all the books in the Lose Weight and Regain Health Series.

Folks with life altering problems like arthritis and other pain syndromes who read the book *Arthritis, Pain Syndromes, and Feeling Older Than You Should: Your Personalized Path to Stop Pain* will need to go from the first step in the process.

The first step in the process is described in the book *Is Pollution Making You Fat? Stop Toxins from Creating Fat* and then all follow the recommendation found in the entire book series to fine tune their eating habits. This is because of the complex nature of their conditions.

People with these complex conditions will benefit from the outline provided in the *Executive Summary and Workbook*, as will the people who want to maximize their health, improve how they look, and how they feel.

Readers can stop at any of the steps in the process, but if anyone is interested in fine tuning their body to operate at peak efficiency, they must go to the end just like the people with arthritis or other pain syndromes. You should take time to look seriously at how your health is being affected by your eating and lifestyle habits. Then take measures to rectify the situation because you may not have a second chance.

Your health truly is above all gold and treasure. Think about it for a minute and take your health seriously.

You'll be glad you did.

The End

Leave a Review

Please leave a review on Amazon to let other readers know your opinion of the book you just finished reading. It only takes a moment or two by going to:

http://www.amazon.com/review/create-review?&asin=B0CQPWXCRC

Everyone is entitled to their opinion, so please be honest. Your review will mean a lot to me and to future readers. Reviews of books are a vital part of helping readers find books they'll love.

Thank you very much in advance for taking the time to post a review of this book. It is greatly appreciated.

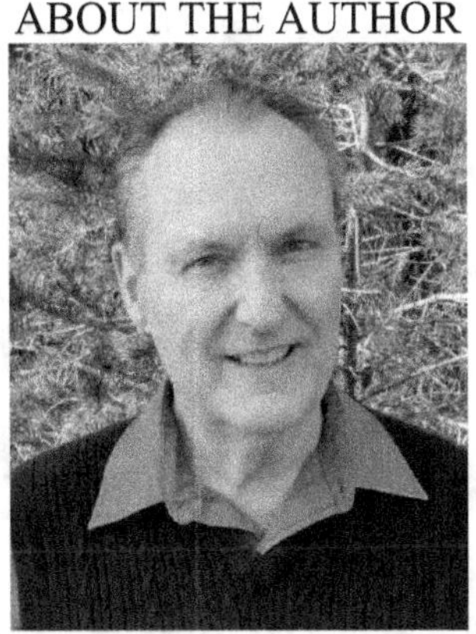

Dr. Heil was born on a wintry day in Pittsburgh in 1956. He received an undergraduate degree in Psychology from Slippery Rock University, spent an adventurous winter in Aspen, CO as a ski bum, then attended the National University of Health Sciences in Lombard, IL where he received a BS in Human Biology and a Doctorate in Chiropractic.

In addition to writing fiction as well as non-fiction books, Dr. Heil recently obtained a Master's degree in Industrial and Organizational Psychology.

He and his wife live in Pennsylvania where they raised their four children.

Do You Like Suspense Thrillers?

If so, check out some of Dr. Heil's by going to WWW.DEHEIL.com

There are a few thriller books there you can try for FREE or at very low cost.

The Psychology Behind Eating:

Scientifically Proven Mind Games to Lose Weight and Keep It Off

Book Two of the Lose Weight and Regain Health Series

Dr. Dale Heil

The Diet Book Series in Order:

Is Pollution Making You Fat? Stop Toxins from Creating Fat

The Psychology Behind Eating: Scientifically Proven Mind Games to Lose Weight and Keep It Off

Foods Making You Fat, Unhealthy, and Unhappy: Your Personal Roadmap to Fix Problems Doctors Cannot

Arthritis, Pain Syndromes, and Feeling Older Than You Should: Your Personalized Path to Stop Pain

Receive a FREE Gift!

Building a relationship with my readers is the absolute best thing about writing. I love to send newsletters with details on new releases, special offers, and other bits related to the Lose Weight and Regain Health Series so we can build that relationship.

Get a FREE copy with email signup of the eBook *Weight Loss Tips* by going to:

https://dl.bookfunnel.com/shegncy941

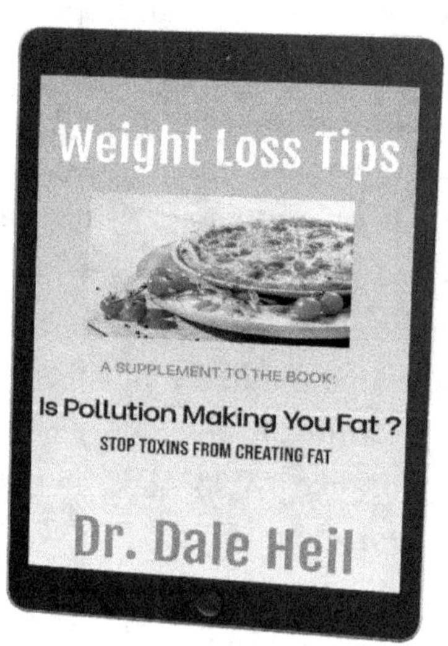

ALSO,

You can get the first few chapters of the first book of this series, *Is Pollution Making You Fat? Stop Toxins from Creating Fat* where I explain how environmental pollution and toxins lead to the establishment of vicious cycles of fat production and how to correct this situation.

That will be at the end of this book… and it's FREE!

Setting The Stage for Learning

In the first book of this series, *Is Pollution Making You Fat? Stop Toxins from Creating Fat* we showed how environmental pollution and toxins overload the liver, establishing vicious cycles of fat production and how to cure this situation. Now, let's look at how psychology can help you get on the right track to not only lose weight or stay healthy, depending on what your goals are (it could be both), but also assure that you stay that way for the rest of your life.

Why is psychology important? Well, let's explore that for a moment.

We've all heard about people who go on a diet, lose a lot of weight, and feel great, but before they know it, they've gained all their weight back plus a few pounds along with their health robbing symptoms. If you're reading this book, you may have experienced that a time or two (or ten, if you are truthful with yourself). Most people have.

The reason you will fail almost every time you try going this route is that you did not know how to apply the simple principles of behavior modification to what you want to accomplish... and you're also most likely eating the wrong foods to lose weight or stay healthy.

This has little to do with your liver making you fat, like we discussed in the first book. It has everything to do with you not understanding how certain foods react with your body.

Since you are now reading the second book in this book series, let me explain how I organized this information. The first book in the series showed people how to stop the formation of vicious cycles of fat production so they can lose weight.

This second book of the series about psychology is necessary because our mind dictates how successful we will be with losing weight and then keeping it off. Why lose all that weight just to put it all back on again? It's what usually happens with people's weight loss efforts, and I wrote this book to avoid that from happening to you.

The third book of the series is entitled *Foods Making You Fat, Unhealthy, and Unhappy: Your Personal Roadmap to Fix Problems Doctors Cannot.* If your goal is only to lose weight and keep it off, the first two books are enough for you. I wrote this third book for people who want to be as healthy as they can be, or those who have terrible health problems they want to reduce or even eliminate.

The fourth book of the series is for people who have very serious health issues that are gravely affecting their lives. It is called *Arthritis, Pain Syndromes, and Feeling Older Than You Should: Your Personalized Path to Stop Pain.*

Each of these books takes the reader further into determining which foods they should eat, and which ones are detrimental to their health. I wrote them in a series because everyone may not want to follow the process to the end because they are happy stopping somewhere along the way. By setting this book series up in this manner, readers can get the results they crave and stop when they want to.

In this book on the psychology of eating, I will teach you how to use simple principles of behavior modification to change your eating habits permanently in an easy to learn step-by-step strategy so you can effortlessly manage food and its effect on your life.

To begin this discussion of how to use psychology to make your journey toward a slimmer, healthier body an easier one, let's look at children and the problems they have with carrying an abnormal amount of body fat.

But why should we look at the eating habits of children? Why not get straight to the good stuff about psychology and how you can use it to get your slimmer, healthier body?

Simple. It's because the eating habits you developed as a child shaped your eating habits as an adult. How did you learn those eating habits? Your parents and peers taught them to you. Just like a baby bird learns to eat worms because that's what momma bird and daddy bird taught them to eat, you learned your eating habits from your parents and friends.

Kids learn by watching others, which is most often their parents in their early years. The psychology that went on during your formative years has shaped you in ways you cannot imagine. As we progress through this discussion about children, see if a lot of it doesn't remind you of your upbringing.

***

Continue reading the second book of this series, The Psychology Behind Eating: Scientifically Proven Mind Games to Lose Weight and Keep It Off by going to

https://amzn.to/3XUE9eA

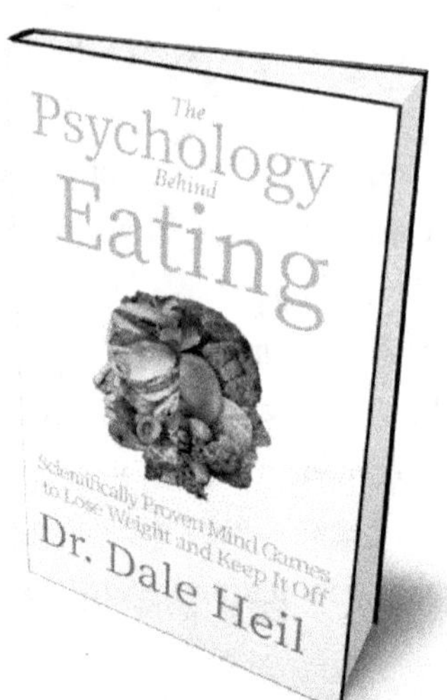
The
Psychology
Behind
Eating
Scientifically Proven Mind Games
to Lose Weight and Keep It Off
Dr. Dale Heil

Is Pollution Making You Fat?

Stop Toxins from Creating Fat

Book One of the Lose Weight and Regain Health Series

Dr. Dale Heil

The Lose Weight and Regain Health Series in Order:

Overview

This is the first book to show how environmental pollution and toxins create vicious cycles of fat production and how to fix this situation.

Do you ever wonder why most people are fat? And why it's so difficult to lose weight and keep it off? This is perplexing when you consider we all eat different foods in varying amounts. The answer is because we all share the same environment. It is the pollution and toxins surrounding us that is making most people carry more fat than they want to.

The chapter on estrogen dominance as a major source of fat production should be particularly interesting to women. But as you will learn, estrogen dominance caused by environmental pollutants affects men as well. Estrogen is often thought of as strictly a female hormone, so men don't see this as a factor contributing to their weight gain.

Then there is stress and how it is guaranteed to put pounds of fat onto your frame if your body cannot expel the hormones that can and will create unending cycles of fat production. And it will remain unending until you take the proper steps to correct this metabolic abnormality. But don't worry, you will learn about that in due time.

Among the tens of thousands of diet books littering bookshelves around the world, none have shown long-term effectiveness. Why would that be? It's because they did not address the actual cause of the phenomenal rise in obesity occurring around the globe. But now, the decades-old secrets of alternative healthcare providers to foster long-term weight loss and health improvements are being made available to the public. And you're reading it!

Losing Weight and Gaining Health

One should eat to live, not live to eat.

- Moliere

You're fat and you're unhappy about it. Good. Otherwise, you're reading the wrong book.

Don't worry, you are about to discover how to change your life in ways you never dreamed possible.

If you're reading this book, you probably aren't happy with your body and need the correct information to help you get it into shape. This is the knowledge you have sought for a long time, and it will be worth the long wait.

The politically correct term "weight problem" does not adequately describe this condition. As a health care practitioner, I prefer to see health-related issues in terms of having a healthy body and proper eating habits or not. Keeping the issue as clear as possible makes things easier to understand. This helps direct people from a state of ill health to improved health by shifting the focus of the debate away from body weight and onto the root of the problem.

Excess weight is just one of the many consequences of unhealthy body functioning. You may not feel bad or sick all the time, though you could be. But what are those unhealthy body functions and why haven't you been told about them before? We'll talk about that, then lay out an easy-to-follow blueprint for you with many options so you can customize your own plan to suit your personal preferences. You will sing the praises of being healthier after you read the down-to-earth approach this book takes regarding health and losing weight.

We will change your thought processes from simply chasing after weight loss to pursuing improved health. Slimming down is just one of the many benefits of increasing the overall health of your body. If you want to be slimmer, get healthier. It's as simple as that.

This book will teach you very simple strategies to be healthier, and because of being healthier, becoming slimmer.

Everything discussed in the following chapters is based on scientific findings and current trends in understanding how your body processes and uses food energy. I will also pull from my almost forty years of clinical practice experience. By working with patients just like yourself for almost four decades. I know what people are willing to do to lose weight and keep it off, and I know why people fail. The information in this book will help you avoid those pitfalls.

Unlike more restrictive weight loss programs, this book takes the unique approach of creating a system that works within parameters you set for yourself to maintain a healthier and therefore slimmer body. In the past, defining these parameters has been difficult. This isn't your fault.

In contemporary society, we are bombarded with confusing and often conflicting dietary advice. "Eat this and don't eat that," doesn't get you any further than saying, "Eat that but don't eat this." It's all backwards and forwards at the same time. No wonder you may be confused.

Many of the weight loss programs circulating around our world are little more than philosophies of deprivation. By basing our discussion on scientific findings and the actual needs of your body, you will be able to sort the junk dietary ideas from the facts. There is some real rubbish out there, and to make matters worse, much of it is solidly entrenched in medical dogma. To complicate matters, the popular media latches onto a select segment of this dogma and blows its importance (and often its validity) out of proportion. That certainly does not help clarify the subject at all.

One of the most important aspects of any "diet" is it must be realistic. Ask yourself, "How acceptable is this way of eating for myself and my lifestyle?" But the truer test comes from asking, "Can I do this for the rest of my life? Or will I just fall back into my old habits and put all the weight back on?"

This book will show you how to establish a healthy lifestyle for yourself. The next book in this series, The *Psychology Behind Eating: Scientifically Proven Mind Games to Lose Weight and Keep It Off*, will show you a stress-free way to use psychology to make it easy.

Since I mentioned the second book in this book series, let me explain how I organized this information. The second book, as I mentioned, is the psychology book. That book is necessary because our mind dictates how successful we will be with losing weight and then keeping it off.

Why lose all that weight just to put it all back on again? And maybe add a few pounds just for good measure? It's what usually happens with people's weight loss efforts, and I wrote this book to avoid that from happening to you.

The third book of the series is entitled *Foods Making You Fat, Unhealthy, and Unhappy: Your Personal Roadmap to Fix Problems Doctors Cannot*. If your goal is only to lose weight and keep it off, the first two books are enough for you. I wrote this third book for people who want to be as healthy as they can be, or those who have terrible health problems they want to reduce or even eliminate.

The fourth book of the series is for people who have very serious health issues that are gravely affecting their lives. It is called *Arthritis, Pain Syndromes, and Feeling Older Than You Should: Your Personalized Path to Stop Pain*.

Each of these books takes the reader further into determining which foods they should eat, and which ones are detrimental to their health. I wrote them in a series because everyone may not want to follow the process to the end because they are happy stopping somewhere along the way. By setting this book series up in this manner, readers can get the results they crave and stop when they want to.

Because extreme diets are not only impractical but also impossible to stick to for years, they are doomed to fail you. The simple changes we will discuss in this book are far from extreme. Then these concepts will be reinforced with physiological and psychological reasoning you can use to prove their worth to yourself. More so than any other diet you've ever tried, this program will last a lifetime.

Oh yeah! The changes recommended in this book will also keep you alive and happy for a long time, assuming you don't get hit by a bus or some other disastrous calamity. This is a good point to remember.

Chapter Three

Why "Diets" Just Don't Work

This is most likely not the first book of this type you've gotten information from. We have all been on the "Diet Roller-Coaster" where you lose weight only to put it all back on… and most likely add a few extra pounds.

The reason for this is simple. Most diets only promote weight loss and are much too radical in their dietary restrictions.

***

Continue reading the first book of this series, *Is Pollution Making You Fat? Stop Toxins from Creating Fat* by going here:

https://www.amazon.com/dp/B0BS4JVWYH?ref_=pe_3052080_276849420

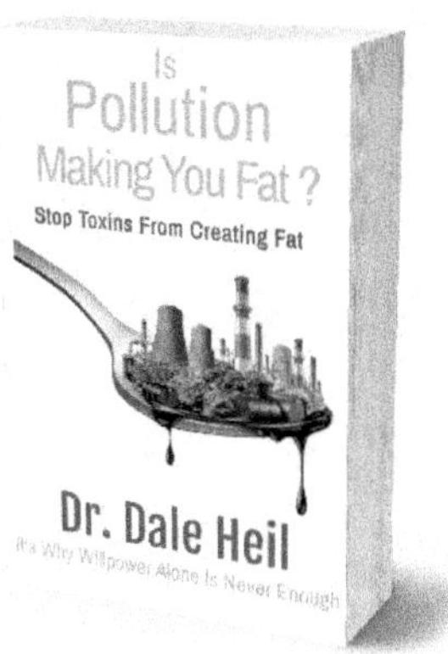